PREGNANCY IN PRACTICE

Fertility, Reproduction and Sexuality

PREGNANCY IN PRACTICE
EXPECTATION AND EXPERIENCE IN THE CONTEMPORARY US

Sallie Han

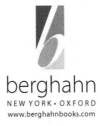

berghahn
NEW YORK · OXFORD
www.berghahnbooks.com

First published in 2013 by

Berghahn Books

www.berghahnbooks.com

© 2013, 2015 Sallie Han
First paperback edition published in 2015

Library of Congress Cataloging-in-Publication Data

Han, Sallie.
    Pregnancy in practice : expectation and experience in the
contemporary US / Sallie Han.
        p. ; cm. — (Fertility, reproduction and sexuality ; v. 25)
    Includes bibliographical references and index.
    ISBN 978-0-85745-987-9 (hardback : alk. paper) —
    ISBN 978-1-78238-792-3 (paperback : alk. paper) —
    ISBN 978-0-85745-988-6 (ebook)
    I. Title. II. Series: Fertility, reproduction, and sexuality ; v. 25.
    [DNLM: 1. Pregnancy—ethnology—United States. 2. Anthropology,
Cultural—United States. WQ 200 AA1]
    RG940
    362.1982—dc23
                                                                2013005549

British Library Cataloguing in Publication Data

A catalogue record for this book is available from the British Library.

Printed on acid-free paper

ISBN: 978-0-85745-987-9 hardback
ISBN: 978-1-78238-792-3 paperback
ISBN: 978-0-85745-988-6 ebook

CONTENTS

PREFACE

Cultural anthropologists study what humans do, including what we construct or create. We make tools and rules, stories and meanings, culture and nature, race and nation, kinship and gender, identities and persons. Recognizing the world as made does not make it any less real. Instead, it enables us to appreciate more fully the vibrancy and vitality of human imagination and invention. In this book, my concern is with pregnancy as the making of persons. Babies (and mothers) are not simply born. They are made through cultural and social practices and the experiences of everyday life.

This book is an anthropological study of "ordinary" pregnancy. It describes and discusses pregnancies that are more or less normal, healthy, and uncomplicated. They are the kind of pregnancies that most women in the United States have, notwithstanding portrayals in the popular media of medical emergencies and reproductive dramas. The focus of this book is on the practices of ordinary pregnancy, which especially emphasize literacy and consumption. In this book, I consider the importance and meaning of everyday experiences such as reading pregnancy advice books, showing ultrasound "baby pictures" to friends and co-workers, and decorating the nursery in anticipation of the new arrival.

These mundanities will be familiar to some readers of this book, and strange to others. As a scholar, my aim is to produce an account here that makes the familiar strange again and brings renewed insight to the study of reproduction. The specialists who read this book will recognize the value of an anthropological study of ordinary pregnancy, which has been overlooked and understudied in the field. Studies of reproduction have been focused on experiences during pregnancy, especially medical and technological practices. In this book, the focus is on the everyday experience of pregnancy itself. As a teacher, my aim is to reach students in the broadest sense of the word. I hope this book will be read not only in college and university courses in cultural anthropology, medical anthropology, anthropology of reproduction, the anthropology of the United States, and related fields of study, but also among pregnant women and their partners, doctors and midwives, childbirth educators, and others interested in ordinary pregnancy and the making of babies in America. I have attempted to write plainly and clearly, to explain specialized terms and concepts, and to communicate and contribute to the insights of the scholars that have inspired and influenced my study. Based on ethnographic research in the United States, this book builds upon scholarship on reproduction, kinship, and gender. It draws together perspectives from cultural, medical, and linguistic anthropology.

In this book, I consider the importance and meaning of ordinary pregnancy from the perspective of an anthropologist, a feminist, a woman, a mother, and a college professor. My training as an anthropologist has given me theoretical and practical approaches for examining and exploring a question, or quandary, that has challenged me as a feminist. How is it possible to recognize both the importance of reproductive rights to women and men *and* the meaning American middle-class women and men attach to a pregnancy? Approaching this question as an ethnographer, seeing what women in my study do in their lives and hearing what they say, I have come to appreciate ever more how we ourselves compose lives of importance and meaning, incorporating even the contradictions. As a woman and a mother, my own experiences of reproduction have made me keenly aware of the significance of pregnancy as the hope, aspiration, and imagination of a child. When I began my fieldwork, my husband and I had been trying to conceive. When a year had passed without becoming pregnant, I went to a fertility specialist who prescribed Clomid, which I ceased taking after several months without success. Then I became pregnant twice, unplanned, during the time that I engaged in my study. The first pregnancy ended in an early miscarriage. The second pregnancy was medically unremarkable and perfectly ordinary. My daughter was born in February 2004, at the end of fifteen months of fieldwork "at home" in the United States. I wrote my doctoral dissertation as an at-home mother. Three years later, I was a new mother again, and a fledgling college professor facing the challenge of connecting with students whose concerns now seemed distant from mine. Today, I not only recognize and appreciate contradictions, but I inhabit them.

In writing this book, my purpose has been to demonstrate the importance, necessity, and relevance of anthropology in the making and remaking of reproduction and of our experiences of everyday life. My intention has been to show ordinary pregnancy as I tell the stories of women's and men's expectations and experiences of it. In order to respect the privacy of individuals who shared their experiences with me, no real names have been used in this book. The names that appear here are pseudonyms. Although I cannot name them here, I am grateful to the women and men who shared their stories with me. I hope that I have been true to them. My thanks go also to the doctors, midwives, and other birth professionals who offered glimpses of their work.

This book is made of the efforts and energies of many people. I am grateful to Marcia Inhorn for her mentorship and friendship. She persuaded Soraya Tremayne and David Parkin, the co-editors of this series, and Marion Berghahn to read this book. I thank them for their kindness, support, and patience. I am indebted to the anonymous reviewers whose thoughtful comments and suggestions made this a better book. This book began as my doctoral dissertation in anthropology at the University of Michigan. I hope it does credit to my teachers, Tom Fricke and Gillian Feeley-Harnik. My thanks go to Nicole Berry, Lara Descartes, Britt Halvorson, Jessaca Leinaweaver, Joshua Reno, Elizabeth Rudd, Cecilia Tomori, and Rebecca Upton for their comments on various versions of the chapters in this book. Linda Layne, Genese Sodikoff, and Claire Wendland offered words of encouragement at the moments when I most needed them.

My colleagues in the Anthropology Department at SUNY College at Oneonta—Tracy Betsinger, Brian Haley, Don Hill, John Relethford, and Renee Walker—demonstrate daily what it means to be a teacher, scholar, and friend. I am grateful to the members of Oneonta Women in Academia Making Progress, especially Susan Bernardin, Charlene Christie, Gina Keel, and Cindy Klink, and to Vicki Howard, Adrienne Martini, and Kate Seeley for their editorial advice and enthusiasm.

Material in chapter 2 on belly talk appeared in a February 2009 article for *Anthropology News* and in a chapter on men's belly talk in *Reconceiving the Second Sex: Men, Masculinity, and Reproduction,* edited by Marcia Inhorn, Tine Tjørnhøj-Thomsen, Helene Goldberg, and Maruska la Cour (2009). Material in chapter 3 on fetal ultrasound imaging appeared in chapters published in *The Changing Landscape of Work and Family: Reports from the Field,* edited by Lara Descartes and Elizabeth Rudd (2008) and *Imagining the Fetus: The Unborn in Myth, Religion, and Culture,* edited by Vanessa Sasson and Jane Marie Law

(2008). Material in chapter 5 on houses and nurseries appeared in the Fall 2010 issue of *Phoebe: Gender and Cultural Critiques.*

This book is based on ethnographic research that I conducted with the support of the Alfred P. Sloan Foundation, which I received through the Center for the Ethnography of Everyday Life at the University of Michigan. I am grateful also to the Rackham School of Graduate Studies and the Department of Anthropology at the University of Michigan.

Sabrina Antrosio and Samuel Antrosio remind me every day of the vibrancy and vitality of human imagination and invention. This book is for their father and my husband, partner, and colleague, Jason Antrosio.

LIST OF ILLUSTRATIONS

Figures

Introduction

ORDINARY PREGNANCY

The joke goes that you cannot be a little bit pregnant—either you are or you are not. Yet, among the women whom I came to know during my fieldwork in the United States, there seemed to be various degrees of acceptance of and attachment to a pregnancy—or at least their willingness to discuss it initially with friends, co-workers, and neighbors or an anthropologist. The women whom I call Bridget and Amanda phoned me not long after they had positive results on their home pregnancy tests.[1] Bridget was six weeks along, she told me, and waiting excitedly for her first prenatal visit with her obstetrician. In contrast, I first met Rebecca and Kerri when they were five months pregnant. Rebecca had shared her news with family members and friends, but remained silent on the topic with her co-workers until the physical changes in her body became obvious. As a first-time mother, her belly did not begin to show until after the fifth month. Kerri, too, was careful about whom she told, not making the news public until she had received the results of the amniocentesis that had been performed at fifteen weeks, then seen the baby at her twenty-week ultrasound scan. At nineteen weeks, Dana had accepted the biological fact of her pregnancy, but left open the question of her emotional attachment to it. "It's still not like a baby to me yet," she told me. "It's a little thing inside, that's all." When I asked whether she ever "talked" to her belly, however, Dana became teary-eyed and hesitant with her words. "I think maybe that's when I imagine it as a baby—a future baby," she said.

In the United States today, acceptance of and attachment to a pregnancy are regarded as normal, in fact natural and necessary. There is an understanding that to *feel* something about a pregnancy is to feel something for the child it is expected to produce, and that pregnant women ought to act as expectant mothers who instinctively share special bonds with—in a word, *love*—their expected children. However, scholars remind us that "mothering occurs within specific social contexts that vary in terms of material and cultural resources and constraints" (Glenn 1994: 3), and that the ideas and practices of motherhood and mothering have varied historically and across cultures and societies (DeLoache and Gottlieb 2000; Walks and McPherson 2011). They even have questioned the "nature" of mother love (Scheper-Hughes 1992). In this book, which is based on an anthropological study of pregnancy in the United States, I suggest that acceptance and attachment represent not where women necessarily start in their pregnancies, but a point at which they might arrive—at six weeks, like Bridget, or almost six months, like Rebecca. Acceptance and attachment do not emerge entirely from Mother Nature and maternal instinct, but become made over time and through cultural and social practices. Or as Nancy Scheper-Hughes has asserted, "Mother love is anything *other* than natural and instead represents a matrix of images, meanings, sentiments, and practices that are everywhere socially and culturally produced" (1992: 341).

My aim here is to move beyond the current terms of American discourse on reproduction. Feminist scholars have observed that as the terms used to describe reproduction have become increasingly restricted, the discussion itself becomes especially contentious. Scholarship that explores and expands the terms and concepts of reproduction is not only an academic exercise, but also potentially an important and necessary intervention into the public expectations and private experiences of American women and men. Notably, any ambiguity surrounding the status of a pregnancy or feeling of ambivalence toward it tends to be regarded as problematic or even pathological in the United States today. Women who do not feel appropriately become labeled "bad" mothers and become subject to the social policing of their behavior (and even to legal prosecution). Jane Taylor McDonnell has observed that "the worst mother in twentieth-century psychological literature is quite possibly the mother of the autistic or schizophrenic child. These two conditions, now widely accepted as neurological (autism) or biochemical (schizophrenia) in origin, were once conflated, and both were thought to be psychogenic, caused by bad mothers" who apparently did not have the appropriate feelings for their children (1998: 223). Indeed, psychologists continue to describe being "unwanted" as a risk factor for so-called attachment disorders in children (Wilson 2001: 43) and posit the impact of prenatal attachment on women's health-related behaviors during and after pregnancy (Laxton-Kane and Slade 2002).[2]

"Wantedness" is measured by medical professionals in terms of the *intention status* of a pregnancy, which is a critical concern because unintended pregnancy is associated with inadequate prenatal care, proscribed activities such as smoking and drinking during pregnancy, and low birth weight and poorer health outcomes in children. However, intention status can be difficult to determine because clinicians and researchers and women themselves do not necessarily agree on how to define it. A 1999 study published in the *Journal of Family Practice* found that what distinguishes "intended" and "planned" pregnancies is the social relations surrounding a woman. "Planned" pregnancy entailed "having a secure job or making sure partner has a secure job" and "having a stable relationship, particularly marriage" (Fischer et al. 1999: 117). This confirms that intention status cannot be understood as strictly about whether a woman feels appropriately about a pregnancy. Indeed, the intention status of pregnancy is linked to socioeconomic status in the United States, with higher rates of unintended pregnancy reported among low-income women. The Oklahoma Pregnancy Risk Assessment Monitoring System found that "among low-income women, 44 percent have unintended pregnancies and 13 percent have pregnancies that are unwanted" (Strong 2000: 172).

Yet, health education campaigns about smoking, drinking, and other behaviors concerning pregnancy attend not to the social context and conditions in which women become pregnant, but to the behaviors and bodies of the women themselves (Oaks 2001; Armstrong 2003). "Women who do not demonstrate proper 'maternal nature,' or the supposedly innate qualities of nurturance and self-sacrifice, are popularly portrayed as deviant and therefore subject to social control" (Oaks 2001: 2–3). The policing of pregnancy extends now to criminal prosecution. In the decades following the US Supreme Court's decision to protect access to medical abortion in 1973, laws on alcohol and other drug consumption during pregnancy have been enacted in thirty-three states and the District of Columbia (Oaks 2001). Since 2006, sixty women in Alabama have been charged with the chemical endangerment of a child—including women who had used drugs during their pregnancies, thereby exposing an "unborn child," which the state appeals court has ruled is covered by the law (Calhoun 2012).

From the perspective of medicine, bad mothers might have preexisting psychological disorders that then interfere with their ability to develop what is considered appropriate attachment to their pregnancies (for which they require treatment) or they might be ill-informed about the consequences of their bad feelings and behavior (for which they require education). Or from the perspective of the law, bad mothers pose a danger to society and ought to be prosecuted. In all cases, it is assumed that sentiment should emerge from instinct and protect and promote the health and well-being of an expectant mother and, especially, her expected child.

It is striking that in the United States today, acceptance of and attachment to a pregnancy—and to a child it might or might not produce—are regarded as natural and normal. Pregnancy and its "end" in the birth of a living child are treated as more or less known and given, despite the evidence that American women themselves could present from their own lives. Almost half of all pregnancies in the United States are unintended (and half of these conceived while the women were using contraceptives), and for every four live births, there is one elective abortion and one miscarriage or pregnancy loss (Layne 2003: 11). In fact, most women in my study did not have their first prenatal visits until the twelfth week. Doctors and midwives explained to me that they did not schedule appointments earlier because miscarriages in the first few weeks are not uncommon. While 15 to 20 percent of known or recognized pregnancies end in miscarriage, it is estimated that the overall rate of pregnancy loss might be as high as 75 percent (Petrozza and Berin 2011).

Historically and cross-culturally, ambiguity and ambivalence, not acceptance and attachment, have been normal for pregnancy. For earlier generations of women, the cessation of the monthly period and other changes in the body (such as sensitivity in the breasts) were symptoms that *suggested* pregnancy, but confirmation came only with the birth of a living human child. "Well into the eighteenth century," historian Barbara Duden tells us, "conception and pregnancy were an ambiguous stage in a woman's somatic experience" (1999: 14). The first feelings of movement in the abdomen, called quickening, were accorded with special significance as a sign of pregnancy and, according to Christian tradition dating to the Middle Ages, the moment of ensoulment, in which a human spirit comes to animate a human body. Uncertainty has surrounded both the physiological condition of a pregnancy and the contents of a woman's womb. Duden, inferring from German women's accounts of childbearing in the eighteenth century, explains that it was possible for a woman to have a "true" pregnancy, which produced a child—or a "false" pregnancy, which did not. The eighteenth-century physician Wilhelm Gottfried von Ploucquet contended, "Not everything that comes from the birth parts of a woman is a human" (Duden 1999: 13). Anthropologist Roseanne Cecil (1996) observes that at other times and in other places, the loss of a pregnancy—which can include what we commonly call miscarriage in addition to elective abortion—has not necessarily signified the loss of a human child. Lynn Morgan (1997), conducting fieldwork in the Andean highlands of Ecuador during the 1980s, spoke with indigenous women who described not babies or fetuses in their bellies, but *criaturas* or creatures. In the Brazilian shantytown where Scheper-Hughes studied, "a high expectancy of child death is a powerful shaper of maternal thinking and practice as evidenced, in particular, in delayed attachment to infants sometimes thought of as temporary household 'visitors'" (1992: 340).

"When does life begin" has been regarded as a question of philosophy, religion, and sciences, but as Morgan (2006[1990]) demonstrates, it is also a question of cultural and social practice that anthropologists are well positioned to answer. The expectation in the United States today that pregnant women ought to feel acceptance and attachment—that is, love as mothers should—is based on the assumed certainty that they are pregnant with babies or fetuses. Yet, an ethnographic account of pregnancy reveals that the beginning of life—at conception, at birth, or at another point in between—remains a point of contention not only in American discourse on reproduction, but also in the everyday lives of pregnant women themselves. Across cultures and societies, Morgan notes, biological birth has been distinguished from social birth. One, a physiological event, brings human animals into the world. The other, a cultural and social process involving both ritual and the experiences of everyday life, brings human persons into a community. In this book, I suggest that pregnancy, like birth, ought to be recognized as both biological and social. I argue that pregnancy is a period of social gestation during which both babies and mothers become constructed through everyday experiences.

Based on more than fifteen months of ethnographic research, this book is an account of what I will call ordinary pregnancy in America—that is, the medically unremarkable pregnancies that most women in the United States today have and the everyday experiences that mark a significant number of them. In this book, I consider the significance of ordinary practices of pregnancy such as reading advice books, talking to the belly, seeing the "baby" at the twenty week sonogram, provisioning the house and nursery, and receiving and giving gifts at baby showers. I suggest that the importance and meaningfulness of the practices considered here lie in their ordinariness, both in the sense that they occupy pregnant women's daily lives and that they represent abilities and attributes regarded as fundamental to human persons. The latter is a particular dimension of the "ordinary" that I intend to develop in the chapters ahead. Scholars and artists long have been preoccupied with what it means to be human persons. Philosophers have located personhood in the mind, and more recently, cognitive scientists in the brain. Anthropologists have regarded being a human person as a kind of habit that becomes learned and taught through experiences of everyday life. As a habit cultivated from birth, being a person becomes taken for granted as natural. However, what defines persons is that they are culturally intelligible and socially recognized members of a human community. This is also a kind of habit, and I argue that it becomes formed even before birth through the ordinary practices of pregnancy considered here. For American middle-class women and men, they significantly emphasize language and material culture, and especially literacy and consumption. The practices of ordinary pregnancy—whether reading Dr. Seuss aloud to the belly or opening gifts for the baby at a shower—are meaningful to expectant parents because they make a baby "real" and "present" to them. As I describe and discuss in chapters 1 and 2, this is especially so during the first weeks and months of pregnancy, when an expected child is unavailable to seeing, hearing, touching, and other means of perceiving that make a person real and present to us.

In this introduction, I consider the importance and meaning of the ordinary and especially what its study might contribute to the anthropology of reproduction. I suggest that ordinariness offers a methodological and theoretical framework to reorient studies of reproduction, which have been conceptualized primarily in terms of medicalization, technologization, and disruption, as I discuss below. Yet, I am aware of the problems that the concept of the ordinary also presents. Who—and what—is ordinary? The account that I offer here is about ordinary pregnancy, and more particularly it is about pregnancy as it was experienced among educated, middle-class American women, most of them married and most of them white. While typically cast in popular discourse as "ordinary" Americans, they are arguably not ordinary at all. The birth rate for unmarried women has been rising, accounting for four in ten births in the United States in 2007 (Ventura 2009). More than half of children born in the United States now are identified as racial and ethnic "minorities" (Tavernise 2012). I am myself the US-born daughter of Korean immigrants and the mother of two children who can claim to be both Asian and white.

Offering an account of ordinary pregnancy that is based primarily on the experiences of women who are white, married, and middle class is a problem not only in that the sample might not represent what actually is ordinary, but also in that it runs the risk of reinforcing an ideology of "good" motherhood that excludes black women, unmarried women, lesbian women, and poor women (Mullings 1995; Roberts 1997; Bridges 2011; Moore 2011; Lewin 1993; Solinger 2005). Sociologist Sharon Hays has noted an ideology of intensive mothering that is promulgated in advice literature, urging women in the United States "to expend a tremendous amount of time, energy, and money in raising their children" (Hays 1996: x). The practices of ordinary pregnancy that I discuss in this book—like the ideal-type of parenting that Hays describes—emphasize literacy and consumption, which can both exclude and include who and what is defined as ordinary. As historians Molly Ladd-Taylor and Lauri Umansky (1998) have observed, "throughout the twentieth-century, the label of 'bad' mother has been applied to far more women than those whose actions would warrant the name. By virtue of race, class, age, marital status, sexual orientation, and numerous other factors, millions of American mothers have been deemed substandard" (Ladd-Taylor and Umansky 1998: 2). Indeed, ordinary pregnancy must be understood in terms of what Faye Ginsburg and Rayna Rapp called stratified reproduction or "the power relations by which some categories of people are empowered to nurture and reproduce, while others are disempowered" (1995: 3).

In other words, whoever—and whatever—the ordinary is, it is *made* to be ordinary. To call something or someone ordinary is not simply to describe what is. It is also to make a claim about the way things or people are or even ought to be. In this book, I make the claim that although the women in my study are not representative of *all* pregnant women in the United States, they represent *an* experience that is important and necessary to investigate. They represent an ideal-type that informs widely held expectations about what an ordinary pregnancy is and the contexts and conditions in which it becomes lived.

Ordinary Pregnancy

As an ethnographic account of ordinary pregnancy, this book addresses a topic that has been overlooked and understudied for too long. There are many more pregnancies than there are births. More women will become pregnant than give birth. Women spend much

more time in pregnancy than in birth. While human biological gestation runs approximately forty weeks, parturition itself requires only
hours or even minutes. Yet, pregnancy in and of itself has received
surprisingly little notice in both popular and scholarly discourse on
reproduction. In general, there has been more concern with birth
and other medical dramas.

Israeli anthropologist Tsipy Ivry observes that anthropology "has
been hesitant to take up pregnancy as a meaningful unit of analysis,
let alone its focus" (2010: 5). Anthropologists have produced scores
of studies on the biological and social drama that is childbirth and
even on the spectacle of the couvade, in which men participate in
rituals associated with women, childbearing, and childbirth.[3] In addition, a body of work that draws from medical historians (Leavitt
1986; Wertz and Wertz 1989) is devoted to the impacts of medicine,
science, and technology on reproduction, which I discuss further
below. When I initiated my research, in 2002, Emily Martin's *The
Woman in the Body* and Robbie Davis-Floyd's *Birth as an American Rite
of Passage* already had been established as "classic" studies in the
anthropology of reproduction. In both works, however, scant attention is given to pregnancy. Martin (1992[1987]) examined the
use of metaphors and images of production (like machines, factories, and assembly lines) to describe menstruation, menopause, and
birth, but not pregnancy. Davis-Floyd, drawing on the ritual analysis of Victor Turner, outlined what she described as a one-year-long
pregnancy/childbirth rite of passage that begins with the "very first
flutterings of conscious awareness of the possibility of pregnancy"
(1992: 22) and then "ends gradually during the newborn's first few
months of life" (41) in the first chapter of her book.

In her work, Ivry discusses the significance of "normal" pregnancy, which she describes as "typically a pregnancy conceived by
women in their twenties or thirties via a heterosexual relationship
and without medical intervention, and proceeding without any particular indications of health complications for the pregnant woman
or the fetus, a pregnancy that many medical practitioners would
categorize as 'low-risk'" (2010: 5). Although "normal" pregnancy is
what most women experience, the focus of public and scholarly
attention has been on reproductive drama. Miscarriages, gamete
donation, and medical miracles that can "save" or create babies become featured in both news reports and the plotlines of television
shows. Even popular advice literature, which is intended for "every" woman, seems to include an inordinate amount of information about the possible problems of pregnancy. "Now that you no

longer have to worry about what the result of the pregnancy test will be, you're sure to come up with a whole new set of concerns," write the authors of the pregnancy advice book, *What to Expect When You're Expecting* (Eisenberg et al. 1996[1984]: 18). The book then presents a litany of worries for the reader, starting with topics such as "Your Gynecological History," "Having a Baby after 35," and "Genetic Problems."

Ivry cautions that "technologies of procreation, such as assisted conception and prenatal diagnosis, are becoming the ultimate perspectives from which to theorize the meaning of pregnancy" (2010: 5). Anthropologists have produced incisive accounts of infertility and in vitro fertilization (Inhorn 1994, 2003; Becker 2000) and gestational surrogacy (Ragone 1994; Teman 2010), and of medical experiences *during* pregnancy, such as amniocentesis (Rapp 1999) and fetal ultrasound imaging (Mitchell 2001; Taylor 2008). Recent work also examines the movements for midwifery and home birth in North America that have emerged in response to the intense medicalization and technologization of childbearing and childbirth (MacDonald 2007; Craven 2010; Klassen 2001). Their work contributes to a larger field of feminist scholarship on reproduction that problematizes the nature of motherhood and of biological reproduction, and illuminates the ethical, moral, and practical dilemmas that medical and technological invention does not resolve but instead intensifies and even produces (Thompson 2007; Markens 2007).

Necessary and important as work like this is, the topic of pregnancy itself also requires attention. Philosopher Rebecca Kukla observes that scholars have spent "vastly less theoretical time analyzing the impact of these same rituals and practices on 'normal' pregnancies, in which the fetus appears to be healthy and the mother has already made or simply presumed the decision to bring the pregnancy to term and keep the child" (2005: 110). She contends the focus on what she calls "problematic" or "exceptional" pregnancies both skews our understanding of the social reality of pregnancy and implies that "healthy, accepted, normal pregnancies are somehow immune from the constitutive power of rhetoric, ideology, and politics and unmarked by social practices and meanings, or that they form an innocent or 'natural' terrain where no ethical and rhetorical interrogation is required" (2005: 110).

A fuller treatment of pregnancy seems overdue. In order to counter the popular and scholarly orientation toward the extraordinary in reproduction and to deemphasize the medicalized and technologized meanings attached to "normal" pregnancy, I consider the significance of *ordinary* pregnancy in this book. Here, I develop an understanding of pregnancy that is ordinary in the sense also that women (and men) make sense and meaning of it through their engagement in everyday, quotidian, and mundane practices. In the United States, the practices of ordinary pregnancy include reading pregnancy advice books, showing ultrasound "baby pictures" to friends and co-workers, and decorating the nursery in anticipation of the new arrival, which I describe and discuss in this book. I argue that these imponderabilia of pregnancy are important and meaningful work in the making of babies and of mothers.

Ordinary Technology

Although my aim here is to move beyond the discussion of medicalization and especially technologization that has dominated recent studies of reproduction, it must be acknowledged that the ordinary practices of pregnancy in the United States now include the uses of reproductive technologies, which feminist scholars during the 1970s and 1980s had foreseen would have profound effects. In this section, I consider the home pregnancy test as an example of the use of technology as a practice of ordinary pregnancy.

Women's expectations and experiences of reproduction have altered significantly in the last thirty years, but not necessarily as had been predicted. Responding to the emergence of amniocentesis, fetal ultrasound imaging, and other prenatal diagnostic testing, an earlier generation of feminist scholars observed that technologically derived information had begun to supplant the significance of women's own bodily experience (Oakley 1984; Petchesky 1987). In this context, they feared that pregnancy would become increasingly "tentative." Sociologist Barbara Katz Rothman described "the specific, heightened anxiety of the waiting period" (for the results of amniocentesis) and "the anxiety generated by the destruction of traditional means of reassurance, the anxiety that comes from not being able to take comfort in the baby's movements" (1987: 109). Davis-Floyd, drawing on fieldwork that she had conducted during the 1980s, argued that prenatal diagnostic testing disrupted pregnancy as a rite of passage because "women experience separation phases that are considerably longer than usual" (1992: 23).

In fact, the opposite seems to be true for women in the United States in the 2000s. Linda Layne suggests that reproductive technologies, in tandem with other changes in American society, "have moved up the time and pace with which many American women begin to socially construct the personhood of a wished-for child" (2003: 17). Far from pregnancy becoming more tentative, there appears to be even less tolerance for ambiguity and ambivalence now. Amniocentesis, fetal ultrasound imaging, and other diagnostic tests and technologies have become not only routine practices, as feminist scholars had foreseen, but they also have become ordinary experiences of pregnancy. Women have medical experiences *during* pregnancy, but pregnancy itself, whether it was conceived the old-fashioned way or with new reproductive technologies, is not necessarily a medical experience. I was told at a birthing class that pregnancy is "biological, but not medical." This is an important distinction to make because it defines ordinary pregnancy for American middle-class women and men in the twenty-first century.

The home pregnancy test illustrates the revised understanding of reproductive technologies as ordinary technologies and of ordinary pregnancy as biological, but not medical. It also illuminates the significance of acceptance, attachment, and certainty as reproductive imperatives in the United States today. Every woman whom I came to know during my fieldwork had a story to tell about taking a pregnancy test, which has become so ordinary a technology that it seems not even to be recognized as a "technology." The home pregnancy tests available for purchase today are known for their ease of use— not always true of technology—which entails a woman removing the test stick from its package, placing it in her urine stream, then laying the stick on a flat surface. Linguistic anthropologist Uta Papen (2008) reads the use of home pregnancy tests as a "literacy event"— that is, an occasion that is influenced and shaped by the reading and writing of text.[4] Papen argues that the test itself is a kind of text for which the manufacturers include instructions on how to "read" the results. The First Response test instructs women to understand two pink lines as "pregnant" (or one pink line as "not pregnant"). On the Clearblue test, a blue + sign indicates pregnant (or a blue – sign for not pregnant).

For the women whom I interviewed, the test marked the clear start of their stories even when they had been planning their pregnancies. Any hunch or hope of a pregnancy required confirmation with a test. Amanda, at the time a graduate student, described a dream in which she discovered she was pregnant after feeling a sharp pain in her left side. "The next morning in my Spanish class, I had this sharp pain in my left side, and I remembered the dream," she said. "So, on the way home from class, I stopped and got a couple of birth control tests and went home, and it was literally like—the test says, 'Wait three minutes'—in three minutes, it was there." While "it" literally refers to the line on the home pregnancy test indicating a positive result, in Amanda's telling of the story, "it" clearly also referred to the fact of her pregnancy.

The positive results of a home pregnancy test are expected to bring the certainty of a pregnancy to the women who take it. Yet, the certainty of a pregnancy ought to be understood as no less an *invention* than the home pregnancy test itself. Historian Sarah Leavitt (2006) notes that the hormones associated with reproduction were not identified until the 1920s, and pregnancy tests were developed in the decades following. Despite their ordinariness to the women in my study, home pregnancy tests only became available widely in the United States in the late 1970s. Pregnancy tests, based on urine analysis, detect the presence of a hormone, human chorionic gonadotropin (hCG), which is critical especially in the early stages of pregnancy. Its detection is not a guarantee of a pregnancy, much less one that is viable. Home pregnancy tests, advertised as "99 percent accurate" and "reliable," are not entirely foolproof, and can produce false positive and false negative results. So-called molar pregnancies and cancerous tumors (including in men) also secrete hCG that can be detected in a home pregnancy test (Leavitt 2006).

In a recent article titled "The Home Pregnancy Test: A Feminist Technology?," Layne (2009) raises the question of whether the tests serve the interests of the women who take them. She describes the results of a pregnancy test as themselves reductionist. "A woman's becoming pregnant (the implantation of a fertilized egg in her womb) begins a series of complex physiological changes. These changes are multiple and incremental. Home pregnancy tests fragment, isolate, identify, and measure a single element of these changes" (Layne 2009: 66). Layne contends that the home pregnancy test is not only reductionist, but also universalizing. Home pregnancy tests give results that are intended to be read as either positive or as negative— that is, a woman is pregnant or she is not—and "suggest that pregnancy is a single thing. But pregnancies are not equal, even physiologically" (2009: 66). She emphasizes that pregnancy ought to be understood as more than the mere presence of a specific hormone and includes changes in women's bodies and in women's lives.

With "early" pregnancy tests available, it is possible now for American women to talk about being pregnant as the first day of a missed period. Women in my study who had been planning much-wanted pregnancies reasoned that the early results allowed them to be more aware and "take better care" of themselves, foregoing the cup of coffee and not mistaking the fatigue and nausea of early pregnancy as the symptoms of flu. However, Layne questions whether the earlier diagnosis has benefits for women. On the one hand, earlier detection of pregnancy makes possible more and safer options to end an unwanted pregnancy during the first nine to twelve weeks. On the other hand, in the decades since home pregnancy tests went on sale, there has been no evidence of improved prenatal care, especially for black women and poor women in the United States. The Office of Minority Health notes that black women were 2.3 times more likely than white women not to receive prenatal care until their third trimester or not at all.[5] Nor is it even certain that prenatal care improves maternal and infant outcomes. It has *not* for African Americans. Not only is the overall rate of infant mortality 2.4 times higher for black women than white women, but the rate also was three times higher for African-American mothers with more than thirteen years of education than for white mothers with the same level of educational attainment.[6] Overall, researchers note that "the evidence for the effectiveness of prenatal care remains equivocal, and health care and public health professionals are not in single accord regarding its primary purpose and effects" (Alexander and Kotelchuck 2001: 307). "Almost one hundred years after its advent, it's still a mystery as to what actually constitutes prenatal care," obstetrician Thomas H. Strong contends, "nor do we know which aspects of prenatal care really confer benefit to our mothers" (2000: 6).

Layne also has described the effects on American middle-class women, who now "begin to actively construct the personhood of their wished-for child from the moment they do a home pregnancy test" (2000: 112). Her work suggests that the earlier certainty of a pregnancy and the accelerated acceptance and attachment to it *create* experiences of miscarriage and pregnancy loss. What would have been experienced as a "late" period can be understood now to have been an early miscarriage. Miscarriage and pregnancy loss up-end the certainty that a pregnancy will end in the birth of a (living) child.

A result has been the construction of a new kind of certainty— the "chemical pregnancy." Researchers have estimated that almost a third of all pregnancies end spontaneously in the first two to four weeks, even before a woman has missed her period or is aware that she might have conceived (Wilcox 1988). During our first conversation over chai at a local coffee shop, Nicole, a woman in my study who held a master's degree in biology, explained to me that a chemical pregnancy is an artifact of early pregnancy testing. A test initially detects the presence of hCG, but later tests then give negative results or there are other signs that the pregnancy is not developing, such as bleeding. When I asked Rebecca whether she had previous pregnancies, she told me that she had "only" had a chemical pregnancy. "If I hadn't known to check, it would have been a late period," she said. Although she explained that it was "technically a miscarriage," Rebecca said that she had not experienced it as a loss. "We'd only known that we were pregnant for like a week," she said. "It wasn't especially traumatic." Undoubtedly, the response would have been rather different for a woman who had experienced multiple chemical pregnancies. Layne (2003) has written movingly of the grief that women suffer (including her own), too often unspoken, around miscarriages and pregnancy losses. Multiple chemical pregnancies also could indicate other health problems that affected fertility. Yet, for Rebecca, at age thirty-five, the chemical pregnancy was a positive sign of her ability to become pregnant at all. In fact, I heard similar sentiments from other women who, having taken the pill since their teens or twenties, felt they were testing their fertility for the first time. For them, the chemical pregnancy was a new kind of certainty that offered its own reassurances. In sum, the chemical pregnancy provides another way for women to understand and explain what had happened to (or in) their bodies as neither a late period nor an early miscarriage. Certainty is not the confirmation of a fact that already is, but is a result that the ordinary practice of taking a pregnancy test produces.

Studying the Ordinary

"Ordinary" often is used to describe experiences like the home pregnancy test—and pregnancy itself—that have been unremarked upon because they have been perceived as unremarkable. Indeed, anthropology as a discipline has long been concerned with the ordinary or what Bronislaw Malinowski famously called the minutiae of everyday life. Recently, anthropologist Michael Lambek called for the study of what he calls ordinary ethics or "the actual and circumstantial—specific instances of conduct, insight, action, or dilemma" (2012: 4). In contrast to philosophy, the discipline that largely has defined the discourse on ethics, Lambek suggests that anthropology, grounded in ethnography, can "speak to the urgency and immediacy yet ordinariness of the ethical rather than reverting to hypothetical instances and ultimately to reified abstractions" (2012: 4). A focus on the ordinary and on practice—rather than on the extraordinary and on idea—is understood here to offer a more complicated and hopefully a more complete understanding of being (and becoming) human.

In addition, what I also intend to develop here is a still more complicated and complete understanding of the ordinary itself. As I discuss in this book, the practices of ordinary pregnancy make babies and mothers, but it ought not to be taken for granted what is "ordinary" in the first place. More broadly, ordinariness itself must be recognized as culturally produced and socially constructed. Or as Karen Sue Taussig, citing the work of Ian Hacking, observes about the concept of the normal, it is characterized both "as 'an existing average' (which can be improved upon) and as a 'figure of perfection to which we may progress'" (2009: 10). Ordinariness, as a description of "the way things are," is always a *claim* about actual life. It is not always descriptive of the way things are always or for everyone. As a claim that is made about some experiences and about some people, the ordinary carries the power to include and exclude. Individuals experience ordinariness variously—as empowering or disempowering, constrained or constraining, taken for granted or out of one's reach. Insofar as ordinary pregnancy describes the lived experiences of particular women and men, it must include discussion of the larger contexts and conditions in which they experience their lives.

I undertook ethnographic research in and around Ann Arbor, Michigan, between October 2002 and January 2004. In my fieldwork, I pursued whatever opportunities I could to watch, hear, and record in my notebooks or on my digital recorder what pregnant women, their partners, families, friends, and birth professionals were doing in their everyday lives and saying about their experiences. I spent time in a range of settings—taking notes at prenatal visits; observing at genetic counseling sessions and fetal ultrasound imaging scans; attending four childbirth education programs that met weekly for five to ten weeks, then completing a week-long training for birth doulas (labor assistants). I interviewed pregnant women and their partners, recording conversations with a subset of interviewees whom I describe below. In addition, I interviewed doctors, certified nurse-midwives (CNMs), nurses, sonographers, home birth midwives, doulas, and Bradley and Lamaze instructors.[7] I collected and analyzed written materials such as pregnancy books and magazines, which women in my study recommended or lent to me. For both pregnant women and birth professionals, pregnancy itself emerged as both an ordinary and extraordinary moment, as I describe and discuss in this book.

Because anthropology encourages us to ask questions about the differences and commonalities with people's experiences in other places and at other times, it enables us to see ordinary pregnancy in the United States today as culturally specific and historically particular. The method of anthropology also requires that we attend to what people do and say, in their terms, and to the contexts in which they act. Ethnography enables us to explore and examine the significance of the experiences of everyday life. The United States has been significant both as a site in the anthropology of reproduction and as a "field" of study in its own right. The global literature on reproduction responds to studies conducted in the United States and to the body of work that American scholars have produced at home and abroad, explicitly and implicitly drawing on the ideas and practices known to them in the United States. It is important not to treat the United States as merely the context or background, but to foreground the particularity of American culture and society in this ethnographic account of ordinary pregnancy.

During the time that I lived in Ann Arbor, I frequently heard it described in terms of contradictions. Long-time residents and recent transplants alike described it as a small city with small town values, with the advantages and disadvantages of both. It was a diverse and progressive community to some, and a homogeneous Midwestern enclave to others. In terms of the study of reproduction, Ann Arbor was a site of the ordinary and not ordinary. On the one hand, as home to the University of Michigan, it was a center for science, technology, and medicine. In addition to the university medical center, there was a large regional hospital. On the other hand, Ann Arbor also boasted an active "alternative" birth community of independent midwives, doulas, and childbirth educators. I had the privilege of engaging in participant-observation with obstetricians and CNMs affiliated at the two area hospitals and with a practice of independent midwives who attended home births. All of the birth professionals whom I contacted about my study were accustomed to teaching students, but they seemed especially interested in the fact that I approached them as a graduate student in anthropology. I think it both enabled me to ask what must have seemed questions with obvious answers and freed them to offer thoughtful and even self-critical reflections about their work.

Not only were the birth professionals concerned with teaching me about pregnancy, but so also were the pregnant women whom I encountered at prenatal visits in the hospital and at the home birth practice. It quickly became clear to me that they enjoyed the opportunity to talk with an interested listener about their experiences, which in part they still were making sense of. When I undertook my study, pregnancy had fascinated me, personally and professionally, for the same reasons that my undergraduate students give for their interest in my course on the anthropology of reproduction: Pregnancy is part of how we all arrive here and what many of us expect to happen in our own lives, but it also was an experience about which I knew surprisingly little. The fact that I was a woman in her early thirties with a spouse and no children seemed more than enough reason to explain my interest in the imponderabilia of pregnancy.

Although I interviewed pregnant women in the multiple settings where I engaged in participant-observation, central to my study were the interviews that I recorded with a core group of sixteen pregnant women, all expecting a first child. What this sample lacks in size, I believe is made up in depth. I met with the women every four weeks, usually at their homes or workplaces, and recorded more than eighty hours of interviews. In addition to recording interviews, I accompanied women on their prenatal visits and to their sonograms, went shopping with them for baby clothes, attended their baby showers, and met for lunches or dinners. Although the focus here is on women becoming mothers, I have attempted to consider the experiences of women *and* men who have been assumed to be disinterested in and disengaged from reproduction. Ethnography suggests otherwise (Inhorn et al. 2009). When the opportunities presented themselves, I recorded interviews with women and their partners. Most of the women were married to men. One woman recently had ended a relationship with her expected child's father, to whom she was not married. Another woman, whose previous partners had been women, chose to become a parent on her own, with the aid of donor insemination. Except for one woman, Audra, who identified as African American and lived in Detroit, the interviewees were white and lived in and around Ann Arbor.

The pregnancies themselves were ordinary in the sense that they were medically low risk. This is not to say that the stories of becoming pregnant were not without drama. Kerri had suffered a miscarriage, endured fertility treatments without success, and begun paperwork for adoption when she learned that she was "accidentally" and "miraculously" pregnant. Kerri experienced the early weeks and months of her pregnancy as a series of "hoops" to jump, or tests to pass. Over time, however, she described "enjoying" a happily uncomplicated pregnancy, even switching her prenatal care from a group practice of obstetricians that had been recommended for their management of high-risk cases to a partnership between two CNMs who attended women with low-risk pregnancies. Significantly, while eight women in my study sought prenatal care with obstetricians, six women in my study were seeing CNMs. In addition, two women were receiving care with independent midwives and planning to have their births at home. To put this in perspective, CNMs attended only about 8 percent of births in the United States in 2003 and 2004 (Martin et al. 2006). Ninety-nine percent of women in the United States have their births in hospitals. All but three of the sixteen interviewees took a birthing class, which is a rate that is also higher than expected. A 2002 survey on American women's childbearing experiences found that about 70 percent of first-time mothers enrolled in childbirth education (De-clerq et al. 2002). Their participation in birthing classes suggests that as first-time mothers, they were interested in, even anxious about, being prepared for the birth, which I suggest marks ordinary pregnancy in the United States today.

Undoubtedly, it is connected also with the educational and occupational status of the women in my study. All of the interviewees had attended college for at least one year, and many had received postgraduate degrees. In fact, at the time of my fieldwork, three of the women in my study were pursuing master's degrees at the University of Michigan, and Dana, who already held an MD, had begun research on her doctoral dissertation on the history of reproductive technologies in the United States. My research is an example of what Laura Nader (1972) famously called studying up and studying sideways. As a graduate student, I was a peer or near-peer of the women in my study, which likely contributed to the ease and familiarity that developed during our interviews. The interviewees included teachers, a librarian, public health and social workers, a doctor, and graduate students. Almost all of the women were in a position to negotiate, at least informally, some form of accommodation that enabled them to work while pregnant. When I became pregnant during my fieldwork, I managed to continue my daily routine of interviews with pregnant women and observations with doctors and midwives during the day, and birthing classes in the evenings. However, the smell of freshly cut grass could cause my stomach to churn madly; I had no appetite for any food that had been grilled, boiled, or fried; and I not infrequently dozed upright while sitting at my computer transcribing my field notes. I wondered how women with "real" jobs handled themselves well enough not only to continue working, but also to hide their pregnancies until they chose to share their news.

This account of ordinary pregnancy seems to be about women who are not ordinary at all. Yet, in the United States, there is a long-standing connection between being middle class and being ordinary. While it is widely recognized today that the middle class itself is strat-ified—Americans identify themselves as "lower," "upper," and even "middle" middle class—most Americans claim to be middle class, as evidenced recently in the popularity of the slogan, "We are the 99 percent." Class typically has been measured in terms of income, oc-cupation, education, wealth, home ownership, and other economic indexes. However, I found that interviewees identified themselves as middle class in terms of "lifestyle." Even with differences in the measures that typically define class in the United States—most, but not all of the women and men whom I interviewed in my study owned their homes—there were shared ideas concerning education, work, and family, not to mention their faith in mobility, socially and geographically. Most of the women and men whom I inter-viewed—like myself—had relocated to Ann Arbor from elsewhere to pursue their studies at the University of Michigan or at one of the other colleges and universities in the area or to otherwise advance their careers and the good lives that they hoped for, aspired to, and imagined for themselves.

Coming to Terms

In addition to "ordinary," there are a number of terms used in this book that cannot be taken for granted. In particular, the use of terms such as "fetus," "baby," "unborn baby," and "expected child"—and "pregnant woman," "mother," and "expectant mother"—reflects the tensions and inconsistencies of the discourse on reproduction in the United States today. Just as a concern with the extraordinary has deflected attention from the ordinary, abortion troubles any discus-sion of pregnancy in the United States. Rightly or wrongly, abortion in the United States is cast as a debate with two sides—the "pro-choice" side is understood to defend the rights of women and the "pro-life" side the rights of the fetus or unborn baby—and there had been little or no room to renegotiate the terms until recently.[8] In this context, *all* pregnancies have come to be seen in terms of maternal-fetal conflict. This is a characterization that I argue against, calling attention instead to discursive practices that contribute to the making *both* of fetuses and babies and of pregnant women and mothers. To emphasize this analytical point, I use the terms "expected" or "imagined" child.

Women in my study, especially in the early weeks of pregnancy, expressed uncertainty about whether or not to call "it" a baby, but they typically agreed that it was *biologically* a fetus. Fetuses are familiar to American women and men today as facts of life. They have become stock images in science journalism, pro-life propaganda, and even consumer advertising (Taylor 1992). They also carry particular importance and meaning "in the private imaginary of women who are or wish to be pregnant" (Michaels and Morgan 1999: 2). Politically, the movement to promote fetuses as human persons has gained momentum with growing recognition of fetuses as human bodies. Personally, for women who have suffered miscarriages, Layne (2003) notes that ultrasound images and other imaginings of the fetus provide evidence that a pregnancy and more importantly a child or baby were "real."

The fact of a fetus is the ground on which claims for its moral significance as a human person are built. Yet, "embryos" and "fetuses" are not biological facts of human ontogeny, but historical, cultural, and social constructions of "human" and "person," as recent scholarship emphasizes. At other times and in other places, human communities have held various understandings about bodies and spirits, the living and the not living. In other words, embryos and fetuses represent particular ideas and practices about human beings and being human. Historically, Duden reminds us, "only recently has pregnancy been technically and socially constructed as a 'dynamic duality' with a fetus as the woman's partner" (1999: 14). Morgan (2009) demonstrates that embryos were artifacts essentially *created by* research scientists of the nineteenth century dedicated to collecting evidence of what they had conceptualized as the stages of human development. Ironically, embryological specimens become deprived of lives when removed from women's bodies and are in fact dead bodies representing the beginnings of life. Research scientists at laboratories around the world collected "interrupted pregnancy / raw uterine matter" from women and their physicians, chemically treating or "fixing" it to produce an embryological specimen that conformed to the standards and expectations of a field of study, embryology, then asserting its importance and necessity (Morgan 2009: 108).

Feminist scholars have argued that the focus on the fetus comes at the expense of women, who become erased, literally and metaphorically, from the picture. They observe that embryos and fetuses typically become depicted apart from the women who gestate them. Yet, it also might be argued that the focus on the fetus in the United States does not so much remove women from view as bring them under ever more intense scrutiny. Historian Sara Dubow traces changes in American public understanding of the "unborn" from the late nineteenth to the early twenty-first century, suggesting that "stories about fetuses express individual and collective beliefs about individuality, motherhood, and American society" (2011: 9). She notes that during the early twentieth century, physicians opposed to abortion, eugenicists promoting the mandatory sterilization of "unfit" individuals, and social reformers advocating for maternal-child health care all employed the same rhetoric, which "began by claiming to protect the 'right to be well born' and quickly moved on to debate the meaning of fetal life and define the relationship between the mother and fetus" (Dubow 2011: 37).

A concept of the fetus is also a concept of the woman who gestates it. Ivry (2010) notes the contrast between Israeli discourse on the fetus and Japanese doctors' talk about babies. Like the United States, both Israel and Japan are industrialized and technologized societies with developed biomedical systems. Ivry tells us that in Israel, pregnant women are treated as "hysterical Jewish mothers." They are regarded as understandably anxious about their pregnancies, which are conceptualized as risks and gambles over which they have minimal influence. In contrast, in Japan, pregnancy is conceptualized as pregnant mothers' management of their children's health and well-being via the care that they take of their own bodies. In my study, I found that US women talked about both fetuses and babies—and described themselves as both pregnant women and expectant mothers. They shared the perception that "fetus" and "pregnant woman" were more clinically precise terms and "baby" and "expectant mother" emotionally charged concepts. Dana—who had told me, "It's a little thing inside, that's all"—insisted that at nineteen weeks pregnant, she considered herself "a pregnant woman, not an expectant mother." Yet, as I described above, Dana became emotional when I asked whether she talked to her belly, highlighting the significance of discursive practices that contribute to the making of fetuses and babies and of pregnant women and mothers.

The difference between talking about a fetus and talking about a baby is not only the feeling or sentiment that becomes attached to one or the other, but the position that the speaker takes in relation to it. In their study of child rearing and language in three societies, linguistic anthropologists Elinor Ochs and Bambi Schieffelin (1984) observed that *perspective* distinguishes North American mothers from Samoan and Kaluli (Papua New Guinea) caregivers, who were not limited to mothers. Unlike caregivers in a number of other societies—which can include older children in addition to adults other than the recognized parents of a child—North American mothers treat infants as conversational partners. Ochs and Schieffelin suggested that this is consistent with other practices and ideas of North American child rearing, notably the understanding that parenting requires the accommodation, and even adoption, of a child's point of view. In this book, I describe and discuss how the ordinary practices of pregnancy involve a pregnant woman's accommodation and adoption of a child's point of view—an ability that defines good parenting and especially good mothering in the United States today.

Here, it is worth also noting the use of terms such as "parents" and "parenting" versus "father" or "mother." On the one hand, "parents" and "parenting" are understood to include both men and women. This is an important and necessary acknowledgment that men "contribute not only their gametes to human procreation, but are often heavily involved and invested in most aspects of the reproductive process, from impregnation to parenting" (Inhorn et al. 2009: 3). On the other hand, sociologist Susan Walzer has suggested that "'doing parenthood' is a form of doing gender" (1998: 8) and men and women become not parents, but father and mothers. "Parents" and "parenting" implies gender neutrality and even equality that reads less as description and more as prescription. In addition to bringing men into reproduction, "parents" and "parenting" suggest the revaluation of motherhood and mothering as well as of mothers. Feminist scholar Andrea O'Reilly, following the lead of Adrienne Rich, contrasts "the patriarchal institution of motherhood which is male-defined and controlled, and is deeply oppressive to women" with "women's experiences of mothering which are female-defined and centered, and potentially empowering to women" (2004: 2). Linguistic anthropologist Elinor Ochs has argued that "white middle class social scientists' dispreference for attending to the role of mothering is an outcome of the very language socialization practices" that mothers use with their children (1992: 347). Notably, in activities that involve cooperation, women nevertheless praise their children as though the mothers were uninvolved and the effort belongs entirely to the children. "'Mother' is underrated because she does not socialize children to acknowledge her participation in accomplishments" (Ochs 1992: 355).

The use of the terms "fetus" and "baby" also suggest the unspoken assumption that nature always underlies nurture. For educated, middle-class American women in my study, biology is the "real" foundation on which ritual, custom, and habit—in a word, culture— becomes constructed. For them, a fetus is an irreducible and irrefutable biological fact and a baby is "more" than that. Parallel with their ideas about fetuses and babies, the women in my study described themselves as pregnant women and *expectant* mothers, marking their identities as not "real" mothers. As expectant mothers, they believed that on the one hand they possessed maternal instincts, but on the other hand they lacked knowledge and skills that needed to be learned or taught to them in order to become "real" mothers. The distance between fetuses and babies, pregnant women and mothers, maternal instinct and knowledge, and the biological and the cultural and social practices of reproduction becomes closed through the experiences of ordinary pregnancy, which I consider in this book.

The Imponderabilia of Pregnancy

This book is organized into six chapters, each describing and discussing an ordinary practice of pregnancy and roughly following the chronological experience of ordinary pregnancy. Drawing together perspectives on human persons from cultural, medical, and linguistic anthropology, I consider them in terms of the ordinariness of language, embodiment and perception, and material culture. As I discussed above, I am aware of the problems that the concept of the ordinary presents in that it both includes and excludes who and what can be defined as ordinary. For American middle-class women and men, the practices of ordinary pregnancy significantly include literacy and consumption.

Practices of literacy and language become examined with a consideration of reading pregnancy books in chapter 1 and of talking to the belly in chapter 2. Almost as soon as they confirmed their pregnancies, the women in my study sought information and advice in books, magazines, and Web sites to guide them. From their doctors and midwives, they received pregnancy books that included spaces to write notes and to record the questions or concerns they might wish to discuss at their prenatal visits. Baby books were received and given as gifts. With their due dates approaching, pregnant women attended birthing classes, which featured lectures, videos, and written materials illustrated with anatomical drawings and other images of pregnancy and childbirth. Feminist scholars have commented upon the medical and social policing that advice literature enacts upon women, especially as pregnant women and mothers (Ehrenreich and English 1989; Hays 1996; Oaks 2001). However, drawing from the work of linguistic anthropologists, I suggest another framework for understanding the significance of reading and writing during pregnancy. I argue that pregnancy is itself a literacy event for American middle-class women. Literacy, as linguistic anthropologists now understand it, extends well beyond reading and writing. It is conceived more expansively as "a process of interpretation" that is "part of one's orientation to a lived reality made meaningful through the interpretation of text, that is, to written and oral descriptions and explanations of events that are endowed with sociohistorical value" (Baquedano-Lopez 2004: 246). The texts of ordinary pregnancy in the United States today include forms that are familiar, such as pregnancy books, and forms that redefine the concept of "text," such as home pregnancy tests and fertility charts. As a literacy event, pregnancy is not only an occasion that involves the reading and writing of texts, but its importance and meaning become shaped and influenced by literacy practices. Sociologist Elizabeth Long observes that "reading is often presented as part of a whole package of values and behaviors" (2003: 14). In my discussion of pregnancy as a literacy event, I am mindful that literacy is a classed and classing practice, both in terms of who reads and who is represented in the books and other written sources. Indeed, literacy long has been a practice that distinguishes who and what is and is not ordinary. In the past, human societies were regarded as either "primitive" or "literate," which suggests the significance of literacy as a marker of human personhood. Nonliterate societies were excluded from a reckoning of "real" human societies.

Whether defined narrowly as the ability to speak or more broadly as the capacity to engage in abstract thought and communicate with symbols, language long has been supposed to distinguish humans from other animals. It is also, linguistic anthropologists assert, "the most central and crucial dimension" of the making of human persons (Kulick and Schieffelin 2004: 350). Again, it is a practice that includes and excludes. In order to become a competent and culturally intelligible member of a human community, children and other novices become socialized to use language. They also become socialized in other ideas and practices of their human community through the uses of language. This model of making human persons, called language socialization, brings into focus "the ways in which subjectivities, stances, and positions are negotiated and achieved, not given. So in mother-child interactions, it is not only the child who is being socialized—the child, through its actions and verbalizations, is also actively (if not necessarily consciously) socializing the mother as a mother" (Kulick and Schieffelin 2004: 350). In chapter 2, I consider the significance of interactions between a pregnant woman and the fetus or baby in her belly—what I call "belly talk"—as the language socialization of a mother and a child. Experts prescribe belly talk to promote development in children. Pregnant women describe it as form of "bonding" with a baby. Both claims made for belly talk point to the importance and meaning of language in the making of human persons. In addition, I argue that belly talk is significant as the voicing of a child's point of view. Not only is an expected child made real and present by attributing to it a perspective and even a personality—as when fetal movements become interpreted as signs of approval or disapproval.

Belly talk entails not only speech, but also touch and the interpretation of fetal movement. Thus, it speaks to the significance both of language as a bodily practice and of embodiment and perception in the experiences of everyday life. The importance and meaning of bodies, senses, and movement is explored further in chapters 3 and 4. Chapter 3 discusses fetal ultrasound imaging or the sonogram and the making of babies as bodies. This topic will be familiar to scholars of reproduction. However, the intended audience of this book also includes readers unfamiliar with both the practice and the literature that examines it. In this chapter, I build upon the previous work of scholars, then argue for a perspective on fetal ultrasound imaging as an ordinary technology. The sonogram, a form of high-frequency sonar or sound waves that is used to produce images, has become used widely in the United States as a prenatal diagnostic screening, in part because it is regarded generally as benign, noninvasive, and convenient.[9] However, scholarship has revealed the ambiguities and ambivalences that surround this practice. Its medical value has come to be questioned as research shows little or no improvement in maternal and infant health even while its cultural effects and social impacts have been significant, especially for women (Petchesky 1987; Georges 1997; Mitchell 2001; Taylor 2008). Feminist scholars especially have been critical of fetal ultrasound imaging, which literally and metaphorically erases pregnant women from the picture and focuses on fetuses. Especially insidious is the current movement in US state legislatures to impose mandatory ultrasound scans on women seeking abortion services. "Since routine ultrasound is not considered medically necessary as a component of first-trimester abortion, the requirements appear to be a veiled attempt to personify the fetus and dissuade a woman from obtaining an abortion" (Guttmacher Institute 2012).

Yet, pregnant women themselves regard seeing the baby at the sonogram and taking home its picture as a meaningful form of bonding and a milestone event in their lives. Building on the critique that seeing is itself a cultural activity—one in which objects become not merely perceived, but actively produced—I argue that the sonogram is a literacy event in which pregnant women become taught how to "read" fetal images at their ultrasound scans. As a practice of ordinary pregnancy, the sonogram involves the making of both the body of the fetus or a baby as a biological fact and the social relations of kin and family in which it is embedded. I frame my analysis of fetal ultrasound imaging in terms of the production, distribution, and consumption of sonographic pictures to call attention to the processes involved in seeing the baby as making a person that is available to human perception.

Following the discussion of fetal ultrasound imaging and the bodies of fetuses and babies in chapter 3, I shift the focus to the quotidian and mundane bodily concerns of pregnant women in chapter 4. Here, I examine the cultural and social significance of women's embodied experience of ordinary pregnancy as the making of babies and, especially, of mothers. Again, my interest here is not so much in the policed body that already has been discussed in other scholarship on reproduction, but in the "ordinary body" that women themselves described to me. This is the body that endures fatigue and nausea, experiences a loss of appetite and inexplicable cravings, "shows" a pregnant belly, and gains weight. It is also a "literate" body in that pregnant women perceive and interpret their bodily sensations through the texts of ordinary pregnancy, which I described above. Although such bodily concerns have been treated typically as inconveniences or side effects, warranting little serious attention, they were not trivial concerns for women themselves, who sought information and advice about managing the physical signs and symptoms of pregnancy and making sense of the changes in their bodies. Throughout their pregnancies, women in my study perceived and interpreted these changes as not only concerning their bodies, but also their *selves.*

Consumption, understood broadly, is a relationship between persons and objects. Whether it involves books as material culture, the baby pictures brought home from a fetal ultrasound scan, or the car seats and cribs that an expecting couple shops for, consumption is significant in the experience of ordinary pregnancy in the United States, as I describe and discuss throughout the book. In chapter 4, I consider consumption in terms of food and eating during pregnancy, which illustrates how the accommodation and adoption of a child's point of view become a habit of pregnant women's bodies. In chapters 5 and 6, attention turns to what we generally might consider consumer activities. In fact, a number of scholars and pregnant women themselves contend that there is too much importance attached to consumption, with the net effect of redefining reproduction *as* a form of consumption (Taylor et al. 2004). Parenting and, indeed, pregnancy are enterprises that require not only new clothes, but any number of other mass-produced and distributed items. As anthropologist Janelle Taylor observes, "The material trappings of middle-class childhood in contemporary America are legion, indeed, including not only baby carriers and breast pumps and strollers and car sets, but much else besides" (2008: 124). Mindful of the context in which the women and men in my study receive and give things—a market society and a consumer culture in which not all individuals participate equally—I am, as a cultural anthropologist, especially concerned also with how and why the things themselves matter to people. In chapter 5, I consider the preparing and provisioning of houses and homes and the furnishing of nurseries as practices of ordinary pregnancy. In particular, I suggest that the child's needs and wants become anticipated materially in the house and nursery. I continue my discussion of the significance of things to people in chapter 6, which describes the American ritual of the baby shower. Focused on the receiving and giving of things as gifts for the baby, the shower accomplishes important social and cultural work not only in anticipating a child with particular needs and wants, but also recognizing a pregnant woman as a mother.

A brief "postpartum" concludes the book, with reflections from interviewees on their births and thoughts on the contributions that a consideration of ordinary pregnancy might make to our understanding of the lived experience of reproduction in the United States today.

Notes

1. To respect their privacy, no real names of individuals appear in this book. I have used pseudonyms.

2. The identification of attachment disorders is based on the work of psychologist John Bowlby, who suggested the importance of the infant-caregiver relationship in children's social and emotional development (Wilson 2001). Bowlby's "attachment theory" has become the basis of popular advice on childrearing, in particular an approach called "attachment parenting," which encourages practices such as breastfeeding and co-sleeping to maintain physical and emotional closeness (Sears and Sears 2003).

3. The interest in couvade, which is evidenced in the work of folklorists in the nineteenth century, might seem surprising, given the scarce attention that generally has been given to men in reproduction. Richard Reed (2005) surveys the literature, noting the various reasons given for couvade, such as a psychosocial understanding that frames the practice as "male sympathetic pregnancy."

4. Brian V. Street and Niko Besnier observe that literacy "has been viewed alternatively as a technology and as a social phenomenon" (2009[1994]: 52). Critical of this perspective, they argue that "both aspects are heavily constrained, even probably determined, by culturally constructed ideologies" (52) They note that "many agents of proselytization have legitimized their existence by invoking their literacy-promoting campaigns, in tune with Western middle-class ideology which views literacy, and in particular essayist literacy, as an essential tool for 'progress,' 'happiness,' and integration into the post-modern world" (57).

5. Office of Minority Health. "Infant Morality and African Americans." United States Department of Health and Human Services. http://minorityhealth.hhs.gov/templates/content.aspx?ID=3021 (accessed 26 June 2012).

6. Ibid.

7. In this book, I use the term "midwives" to refer both to the hospital-based certified nurse-midwives or CNMs who attended births at the two medical centers in the area and the independent "traditional" or direct-entry midwives who attended home births.

8. Rickie Solinger (2005) considers the history of the term "reproductive politics" in the United States. Christa Craven (2010) provides particular insights into the adoption of a discourse on "rights," especially as it concerns "choice."

9. However, it ought to be noted that scans performed during the early weeks of pregnancy typically entail what is called a transvaginal ultrasound, in which a transducer is inserted into the vaginal canal. In 2012, concerns about the invasiveness of early ultrasound provoked an outcry against proposed legislation in Virginia requiring that women seeking abortion service undergo a transvaginal scan, which opponents blasted as medical rape.

Chapter 1

PREGNANCY AS A LITERACY EVENT

"I have a huge stack of books. I'm probably through a dozen or fifteen books," Rebecca told me. "We've really got a gazillion books that we don't need. They're only relevant to a six-month window in our lives." She had browsed books not only on pregnancy, but also on birth, baby names, breastfeeding, infant care, toddlers, and child rearing. Other women whom I interviewed also bought books, borrowed them from the public library, and received them from friends. "We didn't find the books; the books found us," Kerri explained. When she shared the news of her pregnancy with family members and friends, she received offers of hand-me-down clothing, toys, and "practically a library" of advice literature that described the physiology of pregnancy, common symptoms and complaints and measures to relieve them, and the pros and cons of prenatal diagnostic testing.

During fifteen months of ethnographic research with pregnant women in and around Ann Arbor, Michigan, I visited houses filled with books. Almost all were the homes of couples, as almost all of the women who had agreed to record interviews with me were married. These were the homes of teachers, social workers, graduate students, and holders of advanced degrees, all expecting their first child, who was much wanted (if not necessarily planned). In their homes, which most owned, books overflowed from bookcases in the living room, lay forgotten on the bathroom floor, were piled next to the phone in the kitchen, and stood stacked on night tables and dressers in the bedrooms. Books also were bought and received as gifts for an expected child, and were important both as material objects and motifs in the preparation of nurseries (as I discuss fur-

ther in chapter 5). Books clearly occupied an important place in the
lives of the women and men in my study, representing materially a
particular (and a particularly classed and gendered) way of perceiving, feeling, and knowing that is based on reading and writing. It is
not surprising that books and what they represent more broadly—
literacy—were so integral to their experience of pregnancy.

In addition to pregnancy books, women in my study received information sheets and pamphlets on nutrition and exercise and other
topics at their prenatal visits with doctors and midwives. Magazines
like *Fit Pregnancy* were available in the waiting rooms at medical
clinics. Later, reading materials were given at birthing classes. Pregnant women also browsed the Web, especially when they had specific concerns that were not addressed in as much detail as they
might have liked in the books that they read or disagreed with what
they had heard or read elsewhere. Some participated in discussion
boards and live chats, or read the questions and answers that had
been posted on them. Bridget, a high school social studies teacher,
received free newsletters by e-mail from babycenter.com. Based on
the due date that she had provided, the newsletters were custom-
ized to provide information and advice relevant to each week of
the pregnancy, with pictures illustrating the changes in a pregnant
woman's body and the development of a baby or fetus. These especially interested Bridget, who wanted more than what she considered
generic information. "I pretty much check every day," she told me.

Reading has come to be an important practice of ordinary pregnancy in the United States today. Pregnancy books and other reading materials ostensibly inform and advise women on a topic that is
unfamiliar to them. "One of the very first sensations experienced by
first-time mothers in my study was panic at the realization of their
near-total lack of knowledge about birthing and babies," Davis-
Floyd noted (1992: 31). Indeed, women in my study described advice literature as important sources for educating themselves about
pregnancy in general, on decisions about diagnostic testing, and,
later, their plans concerning the birth itself. Sociologist Elizabeth
Armstrong suggests that prenatal education, including the reading
of books and the attending of birthing classes, "has become an expected—even 'required'—aspect of the contemporary pregnancy
experience" (2000: 587). Although the women in my study turned
to their friends and family members, they also frequently looked to
advice literature to guide their decisions. They sought reassurance
when following the recommendations of their doctors or midwives,
and second opinions when they felt dissatisfied or disagreed with

the explanations given during prenatal visits. Even when they did not find what they read especially helpful—the women in my study were critical consumers of advice literature—this did not necessarily undermine their faith in written sources. How and why is it that books and other reading materials become obvious sources for information and advice about pregnancy? What is the significance of reading and other literacy practices for ordinary pregnancy? When seeing the stacks of books, magazines, pamphlets, and other materials amassed in their homes, hearing pregnant women talk about the reassurance (or worry) that advice literature offered, and then examining the obviousness itself of looking to books, it becomes evident not only that reading is a practice of ordinary pregnancy, but that pregnancy itself *is* a literacy event in the United States today.

Linguistic anthropologist Shirley Brice Heath defined literacy events as "occasions in which written language is integral to the nature of participants' interactions and their interpretive processes and strategies" (2001[1982]: 319). Heath's focus had been on the familiar ritual of American parents reading bedtime stories to their children. What is significant about bedtime stories is not that they instruct young children in how to read, but that they foster a stance toward books as material objects to be cherished and as texts worth paying attention to. Heath suggested that both the ritual of the bedtime story and the love of reading it is intended to inspire ought to be recognized as a *classed* behavior and belief, cultivated in middle-class families in line with other practices and ideas concerning education and occupation. Similarly, I suggest that what is significant about reading pregnancy books is not necessarily that women follow the prescriptions given in them—they do not always—but that it provides words, images, and metaphors to describe and define their thoughts and feelings about being pregnant. Thus, the approach I take here both builds upon and departs from previous readings of women and advice literature, which has emphasized the policing of women. Policing describes how others impose their expectations and experiences on women. In contrast, I argue in this chapter that literacy is how pregnant women themselves come to make sense and meaning of their lived experience. Defined in the past as the ability to read and write, literacy is conceptualized more broadly today as the way we come to know, understand, and even feel about our own experiences—and ourselves—in relation to the texts that we read and write.

It ought to be noted also that the definition of text itself has been expanded with the recognition that texts today are "multimodal," or as Papen notes, "they include written text, visuals and even voice and moving images" (2008: 378). The texts of ordinary pregnancy in the United States include not only books and other so-called traditional forms of print media, but also Web pages browsed on a computer at home or work, PowerPoint presentations given at a childbirth information fair, and the videos viewed at a birthing class. (They also could include apps used on smartphones and tablet computers today.) Not only do pregnant women read texts, but they also write their own, starting in some cases with the monthly tracking of menstrual periods and "charting" of other bodily signs of fertility and continuing with formal record keeping and informal note taking at prenatal visits.

This chapter, then, is about more than reading pregnancy books. It is about how literacy—the reading and writing of multimodal texts—mediates the experience of ordinary pregnancy for American middle-class women, shaping and influencing especially their feelings toward an expected or imagined child. By starting with a more broadly conceived understanding of literacy, it becomes possible to recognize pregnant women's reading of books and other materials as itself a form of writing—not the passive reception of information advice, but an active production of knowledge. Pregnancy tests, fertility charts, books, magazines, brochures, Web sites, medical files, PowerPoint presentations, and videos—the texts of ordinary pregnancy—offer descriptions and definitions that women draw upon when they talk and think about their bodies, the bodily signs that they associated with fertility and the sensations that they associate with the fetus, and the sentiments that they attach to the baby.

Pregnancy Tests and Fertility Charts

Papen suggests that "pregnancy starts with a literacy event—the pregnancy test" (2008: 377), which reminds us that the definition of text and of reading and writing has been broadened. For a number of women in my study, however, pregnancy started with planning, and planning required reading books about becoming pregnant. The title that they frequently referenced (and recommended to me) was *Taking Charge of Your Fertility.* In it, author Toni Weschler (1995) describes the Fertility Awareness Method (FAM), or so-called natural family planning, which is based on the observation of basal (or resting) body temperature, cervical fluids, and cervical position to determine "peak" fertility—that is, the time around ovulation. The book instructs women on taking note of the texture of their cervical fluids and interpreting it as an indication of peak fertility and ovulation. The book is illustrated with anatomical drawings of the female reproductive organs and a page of color photographs of cervical fluids and cervical positions that a graduate school friend browsing my bookshelves confessed she had found "so unexpected that I let out a little shriek and dropped the book." In fact, in the book's introduction, Weschler suggests that her book addresses an unmet need in teaching women to recognize bodily signs of fertility that are "normal, universal, and perhaps most important, cyclical" (1995: xiii). From an anthropological perspective, the book calls to attention bodily parts, products, and processes—in particular, the cervix and its fluids and movements—and ascribes them importance and meaning as "natural" signs of fertility.

The central feature of the book is the FAM chart. The book includes completed charts that illustrate a number of scenarios, such as cycles in which a pregnancy does and does not occur. Significantly, the book provides blank charts for women to copy and complete in order to document their fertility cycles. The grid includes fifteen different items to track and appears far more sophisticated than recording the first and last days of one's menstrual period on a monthly calendar. Indeed, charting could be rather demanding, as Brett explained: "I had to chart my temperature every morning with a thermometer—a digital thermometer—at the same time every day because even if you use the restroom, then your body starts increasing temperature. It's pretty regimented. I had to get up at the same time [every day]. You're also supposed to check your [cervical] fluids or position—how far down it is, and if it is open or closed. So, I was charting all this." In part, Brett's dedication to charting can be understood in terms of her wish to practice natural family planning. She and her husband both had become increasingly concerned with the kinds of additives and chemicals used in foods, which led them to a vegan diet, and this had led them also to reconsider the birth control pills that Brett had been taking since her teens to make her periods more "regular." Interestingly, Brett shared an interest in natural family planning with Martina, who rejected "artificial" birth control (like the pill) for herself because it contradicted with her beliefs and values as a Roman Catholic woman. Both Brett and Martina regarded natural family planning as a healthy and effective means of both avoiding pregnancy and becoming pregnant.

Other women began charting for the purpose of planning a pregnancy. Kerri, already in her late thirties when she and her husband

began "trying" for a baby, had been advised that being able to identify her peak fertility would help her become pregnant. Women in
my study referred to the importance of peak fertility in "timing"
sexual intercourse with their partners. They explained to me that
intercourse that occurred too early or late reduced the chances of
fertilization because sperm were not especially hardy or long lived,
and intercourse that occurred too frequently or infrequently di-
minished the quantity and quality of sperm. The idea was to "save
up" and "maximize" the odds. While such explanations might represent the facts of conception as the women in my study came to
understood them, the particular metaphors and images sometimes
gave me pause. Martin (1997) observed that biological reproduction has been described often in terms of gender stereotypes of male
and female, with sperm discussed in terms of activity (penetrating)
and ovum in terms of passivity (penetrated). In contrast to the "romance" of the sperm and egg that Martin describes, the women in
my study frequently discussed natural family planning in terms of
thoroughly unromantic metaphors of time, production, quality control, and efficiency.

The charts themselves contribute significantly to the illusion that
it is truly possible to "take charge" of one's fertility, as I came to
understand first-hand. For several months in 2001, while my husband and I were planning and trying (unsuccessfully) to conceive,
I also engaged in charting my basal body temperature daily. This
required the purchase of a special digital thermometer that detected
minimal changes in body temperature. It was made of pink plastic, apparently to distinguish it from a standard thermometer as a
"female" thermometer. My husband and I developed a routine in
which he, upon waking each morning, removed the thermometer
from its case on his bedside table, and placed it in my mouth as I
still lay in bed. We recorded the number on a chart, using a computer program called Ovusoft that my husband had downloaded
from the Web site for *Taking Charge of Your Fertility*. (There are now
a number of smartphone apps to track fertility cycles.) The software
plotted the temperatures on a graph, depicting a plateau of temperatures indicating nonfertile days, then a dip in the temperature
preceding a rise in temperatures indicating fertile days. My husband
and I marveled over both the technology and the charts themselves,
scrutinizing the graphs of previous cycles in an attempt to estimate
where or when we were in the current cycle. When I did not become pregnant, I took wry comfort in having produced a "textbook-
perfect" chart.

The Girlfriends' Guide to What to Expect

After (or even before) confirming a pregnancy with a home test and calling a doctor or midwife for an appointment, the women in my study began to seek information and advice. In their quest, they talked with family members and friends. Yet, they also found that turning to other mothers did not meet their needs and wants entirely. Kerri, a first-time mother at age forty, found that a number of her friends were now well past pregnancy, and absorbed with concerns like preparing a child for kindergarten or deciding on whether a child might be old enough to be left at home alone. Other women like Martina and Heather, in their early twenties, were the first of their friends to marry and now to be pregnant.

Rebecca felt that reading pregnancy books "rounded out" the other information and advice that she received from other mothers. She and other women in my study appreciated the range of experiences that were described in books as normal because they felt that they should not base their own expectations on the stories of only a few women whom they knew. This was especially significant when women encountered complications, either in their own pregnancies or in the stories that other mothers told them. Older female relatives told their stories, but described them as out of date. Although women in my study valued the knowledge that other mothers shared with them, they also looked to books and other texts for reliable and more recent information and advice. In fact, when talking with other mothers, women in my study frequently sought suggestions on what pregnancy books they ought to read.

When I asked women in my study what books about pregnancy and birth they were reading, *What to Expect When You're Expecting* was the title mentioned most often. It was also the book that doctors and CNMs themselves mentioned when I asked for their recommendations. Other books included *Your Pregnancy Week by Week, The Girlfriends' Guide to Pregnancy,* and *The Pregnancy Book.* In addition, women whom I met during fieldwork read books on childbirth preparation, such as *Natural Childbirth the Bradley Way* and midwife Pam England's *Birthing from Within,* which had been published recently. "Reading is an important way that middle-class women develop their interest in and knowledge of alternative ways of childbirth," Pamela Klassen notes in her study of home birthing women in the United States (2001: 17). Like the women whom I met in my fieldwork, almost all of the women in her study had attended college, and a number of them had received advanced degrees. Klassen found that they were well read in popular and scholarly accounts of the history, anthropology, and politics of childbirth. These included midwife Ina May Gaskin's *Spiritual Midwifery* (1977) and social anthropologist Sheila Kitzinger's *Home Birth* (1991). "These books played a role in shaping their views of home birth and are as much a part of the 'field' of homebirth as they are tools for understanding that field" (Klassen 2001: 16). Other women also mentioned to me titles like Suzanne Arms's *Immaculate Deception II* (1994), Henci Goer's *The Thinking Woman's Guide to a Better Birth* (1999), and Naomi Wolf's *Misconceptions* (2001).

Not every woman in my study was interested in alternative ideas and practices of birth—like laboring without analgesia and giving birth squatting upright or in water or at home—but I was surprised at how many women I met who used the term "medicalization" as a pejorative and were familiar with the feminist critique of obstetric practices considered standard in American hospitals. In fact, two women recalled having read anthropologist Emily Martin's *The Woman in the Body* in women's studies classes that they had taken in college. Davis-Floyd's *Birth as an American Rite of Passage* was circulated in a lending library that Carol, a former midwife, maintained for the couples that took her birthing classes. Margaret MacDonald, in her ethnography of modern midwifery in Canada, suggests that there has been " a close, productive—even formative—relationship between anthropological scholarship and midwifery and alternative childbirth books" (2007: 55). Ironically, although a project of anthropology has been to expose reproduction as cultural and social experience, MacDonald observes that anthropological scholarship has become cited as evidence of "an essential association between women and nature" (2007: 60) that is understood among midwives and the pregnant women whom they serve as empowering.

Historically, American middle-class women's turn toward literature for information and advice on a range of experiences—from home making to child rearing to so-called self-help—reflects particular political, economic, and social processes, including industrialization and urbanization in the late nineteenth and early twentieth centuries. Feminist scholars have considered women's advice literature critically, calling attention to the devaluing of women's own experience, intimate and shared within networks of female kith and kin, versus the privileging of men's expert knowledge, promoted in books that were sold commercially and read solitarily (Ehrenreich and English 1989; Simonds 1992). Until recently, women were the consumers, but not the producers of advice literature on childbearing and childbirth, despite their knowledge and know-how. *Expectant Motherhood,* one of the best-selling pregnancy books of the twentieth century, was written by a male obstetrician, as were other books now considered the foundation of the natural childbirth movement in the United States, such as Grantly Dick-Read's *Childbirth without Fear* (1953[1944]) and Robert Bradley's *Husband-Coached Childbirth* (1981[1965]).

Today, advice mongers tout not their expertise but their Every-woman experience as their qualification to write books. Vicki Iovine, author of *The Girlfriends' Guide to Pregnancy,* depicts herself as a wise (and wisecracking) woman sharing lessons from four pregnancies. "If any real medical information is passed along in this book, it is largely accidental," she writes (Iovine 1995: xvii). She styles herself (or rather, her book) as a companion for women during pregnancy, ostensibly suggesting a different kind of relationship with readers. "While every woman believes her pregnancy is unique and special (especially if it is her first), she also yearns to be told that she is no more confused, insecure or neurotic than the rest of us mothers" (Iovine 1995: xix). Authors like Iovine and Heidi Murkoff, one of the co-authors of *What to Expect When You're Expecting,* appeal to the emotions and sentiments that they ostensibly share as Everywoman with every woman reading their books. Published in the United States in the decades following movements for women's, consumers', and patients' rights, books like *What to Expect* claim not only to inform and advise, but in Murkoff's words, to offer reassurance, relief, and solace to readers.

Even in its friendliest guise, however, advice literature promulgates particular ideas and practices concerning women and especially mothers that effectively police their behaviors. Pregnant women become advised on what to eat, whether to exercise, how much to sleep, what items ought to be prepared or purchased for an expected child, and other matters of what is called lifestyle in the United States today. Anthropologist Laury Oaks (2001) observes that pregnancy books today prescribe what she calls pregnancy rules, which outline women's responsibilities to her own and especially to her child's health. "The idea that babies can, and therefore should, be 'made' perfect underlies pregnancy advice and the medical and social policing of pregnant women's lifestyles" (Oaks 2001: 19). By engaging in particular practices (and refraining from others), a pregnant woman is told that she can protect her pregnancy and more significantly her child from harm—including the harm that can result from her own anxiety and worry—and promote and even enhance her child's well-being. The readers of *Your Pregnancy Week by Week* are advised that "planning ahead for this experience can improve your chances of doing well yourself and having a healthy baby. Your lifestyle affects your baby's health" (Curtis and Schuler 2008: 1). Each chapter in the book includes an illustrated description of a physical exercise to practice for each week. "Studies show that active pregnant women often have fewer problems during pregnancy, while at the same time *not* increasing their baby's risk for problems" (Curtis and Schuler 2008: 58).

Hays has described child-rearing manuals as "hesitant moral treatises" (1996: 65), which also aptly describes pregnancy books. Modern parenting books promote the idea that "it was a mother's job to understand each child as an individual, to be attentive to the child's wants and needs, and to follow rather than force the child's development. The foundation for this child-centered method, it was argued, was a mother's love; because she loved her child, she would necessarily allow the child's needs and desires to determine her own behavior" (1996: 46). Books like *What to Expect* suggest that a mother's job starts during pregnancy.

In my study, I found although pregnant women were cognizant and critical of the expert admonitions on what to do and even how to feel, they also seemed to find their reading rather rewarding and even empowering. For the women in my study, pregnancy books provided a reality check on their fears and worries. Especially during the first weeks and months of pregnancy, when it still felt uncertain, the books gave women a sense of being pregnant. Bridget had received a positive result on her pregnancy test, but she said, "I feel fine. I mean, I feel nothing." Because she had not experienced nausea and other symptoms of morning sickness that are considered the signs of a normal pregnancy, Bridget said she sometimes questioned both her test results and the health of her pregnancy. Reading pregnancy books and, in particular, viewing the illustrations of fetal development in them convinced Bridget that even though she felt nothing, in fact some things were happening in her body. As Bridget and other women whom I interviewed all remarked, seeing even the generic pictures of fetal development and growth "helped" them to imagine a baby "with a real body" inside their own bodies.

"I read and do research when I'm anxious," Rebecca told me, "so during those first couple of months when I was anxious about things going well, I was absorbing myself in scientific information." In particular, she described reading about prenatal diagnostic testing in order to become educated about procedures like amniocentesis and whether they should have the testing performed. Later, at twenty-four weeks pregnant, Rebecca told me that she read less than she had during the first few weeks of pregnancy. "Maybe now because it's going better, I'm more comfortable," she said. "I haven't been quite as avid of a reader."

Pregnancy books reassured women in my study that the metal detectors in airports do not emit enough radiation to cause birth defects and that the glass of wine consumed before realizing she was pregnant will not cause fetal alcohol syndrome. The fact that women in my study not only read so much, but that they also generally responded so positively to their reading is revealing of their status as educated, middle-class American women, most of them married and most of them white. Long (2003) considers literacy in the United States as a set of practices that are both classed and gendered. "Analyses that conceptualize reading simply as a skill (something like tying one's shoelaces) or even as a medium of communication, rather than as a set of activities and attitudes that involves some members of society and excludes others, fail to take this kind of relationship into account" (Long 2003: 14). She notes the institutions that shape the practices of reading in the United States—from publishing houses to elementary schools—are peopled literally by middle- and upper-class individuals, whose beliefs and behaviors become reflected in the books that they produce and teach.

In pregnancy books, the emphasis on lifestyle as the choices that individuals apparently make freely in their everyday lives "creates expectations of how pregnant women live or ought to aspire to live even as it mirrors only some women's realities" (Oaks 2001: 28). However, it ought to be considered how much of the information and advice offered in pregnancy books is representative of and relevant to the number of pregnant women who are not only *not* middle class, but also not married to men and not white. It is understood that there exist differences and disparities in the health concerns and outcomes for white and black Americans, including higher rates of maternal and infant mortality and morbidity for black women. Yet, information and advice that might be beneficial to them is not necessarily communicated in pregnancy books—which in fact has led in recent years to the publication of books written specifically for African-American mothers.

Although there now are a few titles for men—like *The Expectant Father* and, more recently, *Dude, You're Gonna Be a Dad!*—women clearly are targeted as the readers of advice literature. They also are clearly the primary consumers of it. "Women load shelves with books about conceiving, expecting, birthing, naming, and bringing up babies," anthropologist Richard Reed observes. "The men I talked

with tend to avoid written sources. As another father confessed, 'I
don't read the manual and directions for my new computer, do you
think I'm going to sit down and read a book about pregnancy?'"
(Reed 2005: 135). This seems consistent with the status of men as
the "second sex" in reproduction (Inhorn et al. 2009), but also the
gendering of literacy. Men typically have been depicted as the *writers*
of books and women as *readers*. At the same time, women's reading
has been portrayed as potentially problematic as it diverts women's
attention from men, marriage, family, and home to the fictions of
romance that women presumably read (Long 2003).

However, reading a "gazillion" books about pregnancy and parenting—as Rebecca describes above—is allowed and even encouraged. Women themselves regard it as the *right* kind of reading. It is
not selfish, but selfless reading in that it is not always pleasurable
for the reader and it is undertaken in the interest of the health and
well-being of the pregnancy itself. Or as Kukla suggests not only
about reading, but about other practices of literacy that mark ordinary pregnancy:

> It is part of what makes us count as a *conscientious* expectant or new
> mother that we consume public pregnancy information such as guides
> and websites; carefully document numbers of kicks, urinations, etc.;
> report these results to the proper authorities; have doctors measure
> our weight, blood sugar level, and fundus height at prescribed inter-
> vals; and so forth. These practices of self-surveillance, quantifiable
> documentation, and public reporting to proper authorities are part of
> the regime of *self*-discipline that qualifies our pregnancies as civically
> responsible (Kukla 2005: 132–33).

Thus, the women in my study could fly for business trips or on
vacation and remain unconcerned about the metal detectors at the
airport. They also could be forgiven for having had a glass of wine,
in part because they apparently could be trusted to refrain from further drinking.[1] By offering reassurances like these, pregnancy books
essentially rewarded women in my study for engaging in the *middle-
class* beliefs and behaviors appropriate to and acceptable for pregnant women and expectant mothers in the United States today.

Pregnancy Book Critics

Although the women whom I met during fieldwork typically described positive reactions to their reading, they sometimes found

the material in pregnancy books upsetting, off-putting, or just irrelevant. One woman whom I met at a prenatal visit told me that she advised her friends against reading *What to Expect*—referring to it as "what to scare the bejesus out of you." She had rejected the book after reading a few pages in the book about safety. A section called "What It's Important to Know: Playing It Safe" begins: "The home. The highway. The backyard. The most significant risks faced by pregnant women are not from pregnancy complications, but from accidental injuries" (Eisenberg et al. 1996[1984]: 133). The authors' intent might have been to offer reassurance to women concerned about pregnancy complications by highlighting how extraordinary the incidence would be. In contrast, they call attention to the ordinary risks that pregnant women apparently encounter in their everyday lives. I found in my study that although *What to Expect* was the book that most women mentioned reading, it was also the book that the fewest women favored. Rebecca described it as "paranoid." When I asked Brett, a graduate student in social work, whether she had read *What to Expect,* she remarked dismissively, "Some of the stuff I read in books is so extreme."

Brett reacted also to the tone of presumptiveness that she perceived in pregnancy books like *The Girlfriends' Guide* and *What to Expect.* Indeed, other women with whom I spoke seemed sensitive to the fact that the books not only inform and advise pregnant women on what to do, but also how to *feel* during their pregnancies. Most tellingly, more than one woman I interviewed had recalled—incorrectly—that the chapters of *What to Expect* each included a section titled, "What You Should Be Feeling." In fact, the sections were titled, "What You May Be Feeling," and included lists of physical and emotional symptoms. Greta, a high school teacher, joked also that the book had caused her to question whether she should be "worrying about not worrying." For the authors of *What to Expect,* worry is the sentiment that chiefly characterizes and even defines ordinary pregnancy.[2] "I was pregnant, which about one day out of three made me the happiest woman in the world. And for the remaining two, the most worried," Murkoff explains in her introduction to *What to Expect* (Eisenberg et al. 1996[1984]: xxii). In fact, the word "worry" is used no fewer than twenty-three times in Murkoff's two-page introduction to the 1996 edition. "But although worry is normal for pregnant women and their mates, a lot of worry is an unnecessary waste of what should be a blissfully happy time" (xxiii).

The pregnancy books presented worries that were irrelevant to the women in my study—and failed to address anxieties that were.

Given that half of American women continue to work during pregnancy and after the birth of a first child, it seems surprising that pregnancy books have little information and advice to offer on these topics. Instead, *What to Expect* devotes three pages to a discussion of work in terms of the occupational hazards that it might pose to a pregnant woman—revealing particular assumptions about the kinds of work that readers performed—and suggests that working while pregnant is itself a hazard to be avoided. In the chapter covering the sixth month of pregnancy, a section called "Staying on the Job" addresses questions about stress and its effects, such as elevated blood pressure in the pregnant woman, damage to the placenta, and the low birth weight of a child. Women whom I interviewed did not find this information and advice especially helpful. At twenty-three weeks pregnant, Greta admitted that her pregnancy, so far, had not been the blissfully happy experience that the books implied she *ought* to have. "I've had my share of my worries," she said. "I guess I haven't really fully enjoyed being pregnant." Early in the pregnancy, Greta felt physically ill for much of the day, which presented a challenge for her at work. As a high school teacher working with teenagers who had behavior problems, Greta regarded as important her ability to maintain her calm and patient demeanor with her students. She regretted that she simply did not feel like her usual self at school. "There are some women who talk about how great they feel. I felt really crappy for the first twelve weeks," she recalled. "I'm sick. I'm tired. I have to get up at five o'clock to go to work." Added to the day-to-day considerations were larger concerns, including finances. "That's one of my biggest worries because I'm the primary income earner," Greta explained. Her husband, Adam, worked at an art museum, which they both regarded as interesting and satisfying work, but they depended on her income to pay the mortgage on their house and other bills.

Greta, like other women in my study, had particular reasons for why she felt anxious and worried, not joyful, during her pregnancy. They were not what the authors of pregnancy books presented as the normal and natural instincts of Every Pregnant Woman, but emerged from the contexts and conditions of ordinary life. Pregnancy advice, affirming a particular set of behaviors and beliefs associated with women who are middle class, married to men, and white, excludes the possibility that poor women, unmarried and lesbian women, and black and other racial and ethnic "minority" women ever could be conscientious and responsible pregnant women and mothers. However, pregnancy advice also sets a standard that is difficult even for middle-class white women to meet. Ladd-Taylor and Umansky (1998) observe that pregnant women today—whatever their circumstances—all have become subject to mother blaming.

There is a widely held assumption that pregnant women generally accept the information and follow the advice that is offered in pregnancy books and other reading materials. A result is that I not infrequently heard birth professionals describe pregnant women as "not knowing" or "not understanding" when they apparently did not follow professional advice. At the same time, doctors in particular expressed concern about women uncritically accepting information and following advice from sources on the Internet. In fact, I found that women were pregnancy book critics and critical consumers who also "shopped around" for the advice and information that they needed and wanted, consulting a variety of sources as part of the everyday experience of pregnancy.

After having read a number of books like *What to Expect*, which had been passed along by friends, Rebecca eventually abandoned popular advice literature in favor of textbooks assigned in college courses on infant and child development. "I like getting the full background and the studies and things like that," which popular pregnancy books glossed over, she said. At the same time, Bridget felt that pregnant women were faced with an overload of information and advice coming from books, other print media, and especially the Internet. "There's just so much out there. I'm preoccupied with it," she remarked. "How do people work and do this? It's probably better for me to keep busy doing other things, too." Rebecca and Bridget, as critical readers of advice literature, appear to be responding also to the challenges of managing information and advice, which Oaks (2001) notes has itself become a practice of ordinary pregnancy (and parenting) in the United States today. "Part of being a good mother-to-be is determining which advice is best and then following it" (Oaks 2001: 25).

For Rebecca and Bridget, reading rounded out the information and advice received from other mothers and at their prenatal visits. In interviews, they and other women told me that they looked to books and other texts in order to answer questions about minor concerns without having to call the doctor's or midwife's office or wait until the prenatal visit, which initially was scheduled once a month. (Later, after about twenty-eight weeks of pregnancy, the appointments were held once every other week, then every week after thirty-six weeks of pregnancy.) For the women in my study, advice literature seemed both equally reliable and more convenient.

In fact, doctors and midwives whom I met during fieldwork encouraged pregnant women to read. In addition to liberally dispensing brochures and other reading materials, they were more likely to recommend books than other sources when pregnant women asked.

Doctors also were more likely to express their skepticism about sources on the Internet, which they said could spread misinformation. The admonitions to patients not to trust Web sources—and the complaints shared among doctors and nurses about patients "bringing print-outs" to their prenatal visits—became so oft-repeated that I started to wonder why. The women in my study themselves were concerned with reading credible sources, which is a reason why they brought print-outs to their doctors and midwives to check the information and advice on the Internet. I noted also that a number of traditional print media (like magazines) and even hospitals themselves, including the university medical center, had created Web sites featuring information and advice for pregnant women. It became clear to me that when doctors expressed their skepticism about the Internet, they specifically meant discussion boards where women shared information and advice derived from their own experiences. It also became clear that the information and advice presented on discussion boards were not always inaccurate. Doctors seemed to be cautioning pregnant women about the *chance* of there being misinformation on Web sources. I began to understand their skepticism about the Internet as based in part with their lack of familiarity with it and in part with their lack of control over and even authority within a forum like a discussion board where every pregnant woman can ask and answer questions.

Pregnancy and Record Keeping

Davis-Floyd has suggested that "doctors in this society have taken on the role of the ritual elder in many cross-cultural initiation rites, but with one important difference" (1992: 29). Instead of elders enabling and empowering initiates with knowledge, however, she described doctors in the United States withholding information from pregnant women, using "clipboards, standardized charts, and technical jargon that symbolically shout 'off limits' to the uninitiated" (1992: 30). The keeping of medical records can be understood as an instrument of authority as pregnant bodies become examined, evaluated, then written about in files not open to pregnant women themselves, but maintained in the possession of hospitals. It is in this context that I observed the CNMs in one hospital-based practice make a particular point of showing women their files, at least on occasion, during their prenatal visits. At the home birth practice where I observed, the midwives greeted each pregnant woman, handing her file to her. The woman then weighed herself on the bathroom scale, tested her own urine, and wrote her information in her file. Faith and Radha, the home birth midwives, told me that the purpose of having pregnant women actively measure and record their own information was *not* to treat them as patients with little or no ability or knowledge.

This is exactly why Kerri switched from a large group practice of obstetricians to a small partnership between two CNMs. She appreciated what she regarded as the "more personal" attention that she and her husband, Brian, both received from the midwives. What she more specifically described to me was their "egalitarian style" of "explaining, not teaching," so that she felt "more of a participant" in the decisions concerning her medical care. Other women in my study who sought care with obstetricians also praised their particular doctors for their willingness to listen and to take seriously their concerns. Indeed, most of the prenatal visits that I observed in my fieldwork proceeded as conversations, with doctors and midwives typically allowing pregnant women to introduce their concerns first before offering information and advice.

Kerri and other women in my study approached their prenatal care providers as specialists, not authorities. They expected to consult with their doctors and midwives, not be talked to. The decisions that they made concerning their prenatal medical care reflect both the relative privilege of most (but not all) of the women in my study, who were well educated and pursuing professional careers. Of the sixteen women in my core group of interviewees, six women sought care during pregnancy and birth with CNMs at the two hospitals in the area, and two women prepared for home births with independent, direct-entry midwives—that is, midwives who were unaffiliated with a hospital and who had received training through apprenticeship. These numbers are not representative of American middle-class women's experiences. In the United States today, 99 percent of all births occur in the hospital, with doctors, specifically obstetricians, attending 90 percent and CNM's the remaining 10 percent of these. Less than 1 percent of all births occur at home, and only a percentage of these with direct-entry midwives. In the United States, where births occur and with whom in attendance depend upon access to health insurance, which remains a benefit available primarily through employers. Most of the women in my study had health insurance, their own or their spouse's, which covered almost all of the expenses associated with hospital-based care during pregnancy and birth. Home births, however, were not covered at all. Nicole and Betsy, the two women in my study who planned home births, paid for the fees (which averaged about $3,000) from their own pockets even though both women had health insurance that would have covered almost the entire cost of a hospital birth (which might have cost two to three times more, even for an uncomplicated vaginal delivery).

Nicole had felt that as a patient in a hospital-based practice, she had been encouraged to be a passive recipient of the information and advice the obstetricians and midwives there had given her. She had questioned some of the information and advice that she received during her initial prenatal visits with the CNMs. Having earned a master's degree in biology and worked in a research laboratory, she preferred to seek information actively for herself rather than receive what she considered "distilled" advice from the CNMs. "I never have any questions because if I had a question, I'd look it up myself," Nicole explained. "Not only do I have books, I have the Internet and I have my Web board where I can look up questions that other people have asked and answers that other people gave." Later, she described an awkward conversation that she had when she asked a CNM for a copy of her file. Nicole requested it because she had begun planning for a home birth with independent midwives. The CNM had been reluctant to give it to her, even though, Nicole insisted, "it is *my* file."

At the time, I agreed with Nicole on the point that it was *her* file, but as a cultural anthropologist, I have begun to reconsider whether or not that is the case. The file bore her name, contained information about her, and had been maintained ostensibly for her benefit, but a case might be made also that the file in fact belongs to the doctors or midwives, whose work it also documents. The incorporation of pregnant women into the writing of files might not necessarily be about empowering women, but rather it might be about encouraging them to become more involved in their medical care—or put in other terms, inviting pregnant women to be compliant as patients. Papen (2008) suggests that this is, in fact, one of the observed effects and one of the explicit purposes of the Personal Maternity Record, or "Green Notes," that pregnant women in England, under the National Health Service, are required to keep. That is, pregnant women both hold the Green Notes in their possession, presenting them at their prenatal visits, and maintain them, collecting test results and other documents. However, the Green Notes significantly feature not the writing of a pregnant woman, but the notations of midwives and doctors, documenting the dates of their appointments, the topics and recommendations that were discussed, information such as the pregnant woman's weight and blood pressure, and the care provider's observations about the pregnant woman's condition. As a result, Papen suggests that the Green Notes "can also be seen as a surveillance tool in the Foucauldian sense" (2008: 389), intended to produce what Michel Foucault had called docile bodies that follow the recommendations of doctors and midwives (e.g., on what to eat and how much weight to gain), and comply with the ideas and practices of institutions like hospitals. Of her own experiences with Green Notes, Papen recalls: "At the end of each meeting with a midwife, I could see them writing their brief reports. But they never told me what they were writing. Nor did they check with me that I agreed with what they put. Because of this I didn't feel I had any stake or ownership in the records they produced" (2008: 387). She regarded the Green Notes as belonging not to her, but to her midwives. "As a literacy practice, they were shaped by the needs of the health care providers and the culture of work of the NHS" (2008: 388).

Ivry (2010) describes the meticulous record keeping of pregnant women in Japan. It includes the *boshitecho,* or mother-child handbook, which municipalities provide to women as a medical record of their pregnancies. In contrast to medical files in the United States and Green Notes in England, the mother-child handbook in Japan "is a written manifestation and symbol of *the shared responsibility of the mother and medical practitioners:* it is designed for both the mothers and the practitioners to complete" (Ivry 2010: 142). The *boshitecho* includes spaces for women to record observations about their daily routines, bodily sensations, and moods in addition to information from their prenatal visits such as weight, urine, and blood pressure. Ivry emphasizes that although Japanese women's record keeping looks remarkable to American or English women, it is also part of "a literary cultural tradition of meticulous, snapshot-style documentations" that dates even to the personal diaries of medieval courtesans (2010: 145–46). She observes also that Japanese women themselves appear not to experience record keeping as Foucauldian surveillance, but in fact express pleasure in the writing of notes— describing it even as an opportunity to exercise "talent" at keeping a diary—and satisfaction with the production of a document to have in hand and later to share with a child. In fact, Japanese women describe the *boshitecho* as itself a form of care giving to their children, as the charting of children's habits, starting with sleeping and eating, is recognized as integral to parenting.

In comparison with and in contrast to the experiences of pregnant women in England and in Japan that Papen (2008) and Ivry (2010) respectively describe, women in the United States are not required or expected to write much about their pregnancies. The women seeking prenatal care at the university medical center received a spiral-bound book titled, *You, Your Baby & Us*, which included phone numbers for the hospital birth center and emergency room and information about the particular concerns associated with each trimester. There were pages on which a woman might complete a medical history of herself, and additional lined pages for pregnant women to take notes at their prenatal visits. The book also included checklists that I learned were copies of the intake forms that pregnant women completed and that doctors and CNMs discussed with them during prenatal visits. Most of the items on the checklists were statements that referred to pregnant women's access to information, such as "I have the information and help I need to deal with my emotions and feelings about pregnancy." Yet, the completed checklists were placed in the file kept on each patient at the medical center. In my fieldwork observations and in my own experience, I found that after the book was presented at the first prenatal visit, it was not discussed again until closer to the delivery date. At that point, I was advised not to hesitate to call about my concerns, and reminded that I had been given the phone numbers for the hospital in the book.

On another occasion, a CNM remarked that I had written "a lot" in my book. In fact, I used the lined pages to record my weight and blood pressure at my appointments and, in between prenatal visits, occasionally to jot down a question that I planned to ask, like whether it was necessary for me to schedule a sonogram separately. As an ethnographer (and a former newspaper reporter), I likely take more notes than many other women do—I documented my own pregnancy in my field notes for this study and in a separate pregnancy journal—but I did not necessarily perceive the notes in my hospital book as themselves "a lot" of writing. This led me to think that other women, whether or not they were taking notes, were not using the book to record them. Pregnant women in my study had shown me the pregnancy journals and baby books they had received as gifts from family members and friends. Were they writing in them? I wanted to know. Greta, who still was dressed in her clothes for work, as she had to walk her dog and not had time to change before meeting me to record an interview, told me no, she had not been. In fact, this was why she was recording interviews with a cultural anthropologist.

In addition to the Green Notes, Papen (2008) also discussed the significance of keeping a personal diary during pregnancy. "Writing about my experiences helped me build my new identity and it was in writing that I also negotiated the relationship between new and old (i.e. pre-pregnancy) selves" (Papen 2008: 392). Certainly, writing is not the only or even the most significant act of meaning making available to pregnant women—in this book, I discuss other practices of ordinary pregnancy—but it is important to recognize *who* writes and *what* they write about pregnancy and how that influences women's expectations and experiences in the United States today.

Birthing Classes as Literacy Events

"Is it time to have a baby?" This was the theme of a seminar and information fair that one of the two major medical centers in the area sponsored each year. Some of the women were visibly pregnant, and some made a point of telling the doctors and midwives whom they met that they were just planning ahead. The morning-long seminar featured PowerPoint presentations from obstetricians, CNMs, and nurses at the medical center. Door prizes such as a manual breast pump and an infant car seat—the artifacts of the material culture of modern parenting in the United States—were announced and awarded at intervals, adding to the sense of anticipation that seemed to hang over the auditorium. A breakfast of fruit, pastries, juice, coffee, and tea was served during a break. After the seminar, the attendees—almost all of them female-male couples—browsed informational displays and collected brochures, pens, and refrigerator magnets from organizations like the March of Dimes and the county health department. These were in addition to the three-ring binder of written materials that had been distributed to the attendees.

During the seminar, the PowerPoint presentation that elicited the most audible response began with a brief history of childbirth. Historical images of a woman in a birthing chair and a woman upright and hanging onto a rope that dangled from overhead provoked stunned silence, then laughter as the labor and delivery nurse giving the presentation reassured the audience that "we have come a long way" toward making childbirth "more comfortable" for women. The presentation then continued with photographs of the clean, well-lighted, and medically equipped and staffed labor, delivery, and recovery rooms at the medical center. In the guise of educating women and their partners about a range of issues concerning pregnancy and childbirth, the event clearly was intended also to advertise both this particular hospital as a place to have a baby and more generally the hospital birth as a modern and comfortable experience.

Armstrong suggests that activities like this forum, purported to meet the needs of individual women, in fact serve the institutional interests of hospitals "in an economic environment in which hospitals compete fiercely with each other through lavish advertising, luxurious birthing suites, and up-to-date neonatal intensive care units for the lucrative baby business, which they also see as building a loyal customer base" (2000: 584). Indeed, women in my study recognized that they were being courted for their business. Greta told me that she had attended the seminar primarily to help her decide at which area hospital to find a doctor or midwife. Ultimately, the information and advice that she received at the event were less important than what she described as the "feeling" that she received there. It is this notion of feeling and its cultivation through activities like the seminar and birthing classes—as literacy events that train pregnant women's perceptions—which I emphasize here.

For American middle-class women and men, birth marks the end of pregnancy, and the beginning of childhood and parenting. During pregnancy, women and men in my study described their anticipation of the birth with a mixture of joy, fear, relief, and anxiety as they imagined the new child, their new roles and responsibilities as parents, and their new lives as families. In the final months and weeks leading to the due date, however, the focus of their concern was on the parturition itself and especially the pain associated with labor. Pregnant women and their partners described childbirth as their final hoop, and the pain of labor itself as a test or challenge, especially when they, like Betsy, hoped to have a "natural" childbirth. For the women in my study, a "natural" childbirth could refer to experiences as vastly different as a hospital birth with no pain medication or a home birth attended by midwives, but what they had in common was the conscious and active participation of women (Davis-Floyd 1992).[3] Betsy told me that she trusted her midwives to guide her through a home birth, and that she needed "to trust in her body." She felt anxious about the pain of labor, or rather her response to it. She feared "losing control" of herself. Paradoxically, "natural" childbirth has come to be seen as requiring training and education (Mansfield 2008). Like other women in my study, Betsy sought preparation for her birth by reading books, talking to her midwives and to her friends, watching videos, and enrolling in birthing classes.

A recent survey found that 56 percent of first-time mothers attended childbirth education classes in 2005—a steep decline from the 70 percent attending classes in 2001—and that only 11 percent regarded the classes as a routine part of pregnancy (DeClerq et al. 2006). Midwives, doulas, and childbirth educators lamented to me the decline in participation, which they blamed on the normalization of medical management and intervention during labor and delivery. I was told that because pregnant women assumed that they could and would receive an epidural, they no longer regarded preparation for childbirth as necessary. Nevertheless, birthing classes were a meaningful experience of ordinary pregnancy for the women with whom I recorded interviews. All but one of the sixteen interviewees attended birthing classes.

During my fieldwork, I participated and observed in the five programs that the women in my study had attended (but not necessarily at the same time with the interviewees). Five of the interviewees attended Lamaze classes. It is surprising that more did not, given that Lamaze was the best known—an international brand that is synonymous with childbirth education—and most of the interviewees could have attended at no cost because their health insurance plans reimbursed the fees. However, interviewees perceived Lamaze as "hospital-oriented," an impression that Armstrong (2000) also documents in her analysis. An interest in "natural" childbirth influenced the decisions that women made concerning which birthing classes they enrolled in (and paid for). Four of the sixteen women attended Bradley classes, another nationally known program, at a community center. I soon learned that the Bradley Method had a reputation as "hard core about natural childbirth," which was viewed positively among expectant couples, but somewhat negatively among obstetricians.[4] Two other classes, Holistic and Birthing Awareness, were designed and taught by local midwives who attended home births, and met in their offices. I attended the fifth class, Hypnobirthing, as both a participant-observer and a pregnant woman preparing for the birth of my first child. It was taught in a series of private lessons at the instructor's home.

Doctors and midwives whom I met during fieldwork recommended childbirth education—typically Lamaze classes—to their patients and clients. From birthing classes, expectant parents themselves sought technical information about the terms used to describe labor, like dilation, effacement, and transition. What they especially wanted to know, however, was how to manage the pain of labor and control themselves. "I want to know what kind of pain this is," Betsy told me. "I've heard it's just excruciating, but I'm hoping to try and just cope with it, just deal with it as millions of women have." After a pause, she said, "I'm worried—I don't want to be a screamer. I really don't. I really hope that I'm a quiet one just because I don't want to scream like that." After another pause, she added, "I have to be honest—one of my fears is pooping all over the place. Because I hear sometimes that it just happens, and I don't want that to happen." Laughing, she explained, "I'm sure the midwives have dealt with that before, but I hope that doesn't happen. It's one of my fears. It really is." Other women whom I interviewed were concerned similarly with how the experience of pain might affect them, and how they might "act" or "behave" during childbirth. Men, too, were anxious, both for their partners, and about themselves and their ability to "coach" or "assist" at the birth.

Intended as instrumental preparation, childbirth education classes are significant also as a ritual of American pregnancy. Davis-Floyd (1992) suggested that for expectant parents, the classes are an experience of communitas—the intense solidarity shared among individuals in liminality, or transition from one status to another, in rites of passage. She described attending a class as a form of ritual intensification for women and men to "get psyched" for the birth. Reed (2005) contends that childbirth education classes are especially important for American middle-class men.[5] "Birthing classes, not books or mentors, teach a man about pregnancy and childbirth, usually while he is sitting on the floor with his partner, surrounded by a dozen or so other pregnant couples. Once a week for six to twelve weeks, soon-to-be fathers set aside work and play to retreat into a dimly lit room where they learn the magic and the mysteries of birth" (Reed 2005: 135). In addition to intellectual readiness, childbirth education classes provide for men in particular a space and time for emotional and spiritual reflection.

Armstrong (2000) offers a more skeptical perspective on birthing classes, in particular the programs that hospitals now offer almost as a matter of course. She suggests that although they are advertised as educational opportunities for women and men to prepare themselves for childbirth, in fact the classes are "focused on teaching women on how to be accountable for the hospital birth process itself" (Armstrong 2000: 588). This is a perception that the women in my study also shared, as I noted above. Following the lead of Erving Goffman, Armstrong argues that "prenatal and childbirth services in hospitals are primarily organized and designed to meet institutional needs" (2000: 584). These included cultivating an acceptance of a loss of privacy in the hospital setting and familiarizing women and men with the hospital's policies, such as how long a woman stays and when she can be discharged. Armstrong suggests that childbirth education "purports to teach pregnant women an alternative way to experience childbirth, one not dominated by the dictates of medicine or hospital, but really functions to prepare them for compliance with the institutional regime" (2000: 601).

As anthropologists long have observed, communities enact their core beliefs and values in their practices of everyday life and in their rituals. Typically, rituals are regarded as special activities, removed from ordinary experiences and characterized by pattern, repetition, and particular attention to symbols. They are performed to mark or in fact effect a meaningful change. Involving a community, a ritual, like the baby shower, is a display and enactment of public acknowledgement and social recognition. Rituals also have important cognitive and psychological effects on the individuals who participate in them. From the perspective of anthropology, birthing classes are significant for this reason especially. They teach American middle-class women and men not only what happens and what to do during childbirth—a form of specialized or ritual knowledge—but also how to *feel*. Feeling refers both to sentiment and emotion and to sensory perception. Childbirth education classes train (or retrain) expectant parents in how to feel about pain as it defines the experience of birth. Birthing classes presented expectant parents in my study with images, metaphors, and paradigms of childbirth. Pain itself comes to be defined and experienced as suffering to be eliminated or as productive activity to work with (not against) or even as sensation to be "embraced." For American middle-class women and men, childbirth education classes serve as cultural and social resources for making sense and meaning of their experiences.

"I don't remember a whole lot from those classes. There was just one thing I remembered that they had, this little model of a pelvis and they told us how the baby needed to come through that," Reed was told by a man in his study, "and I was like, 'Oh, okay, I never thought that the baby had to go through the pelvis'" (2005: 135). Instructors used a number of props and visual aids, like three-dimensional models, charts, or pictures, in their presentations. One woman in my study later recalled that the instructor of her birthing class had used a small paper plate to demonstrate the dilation (opening or widening) of a woman's cervix from "zero" (a dot in the center) to "ten" (the diameter of the plate). Visual images also figured prominently in the written materials that were given to expectant parents at the classes as references to consult and revisit as the due date drew nearer. These included books, informational brochures, and folders containing articles photocopied from magazines and Web sites.

For childbirth educators, metaphors and images helped communicate ideas and teach concepts more effectively. Brigitte Jordan (1993[1978]), commenting on why government-sponsored training courses for indigenous midwives had failed, observed that Western, or more particularly American and European, pedagogy relies on visual aids and assumed development of a particular kind of visual literacy. In addition to being able to read the manipulation of photographic representations—"increasing or decreasing the size of the object represented, decontextualizing it by blanking out the background, changing colors in certain ways, and so on"—Jordan noted, "We in the West also subscribe to a set of rules for interpreting line drawings and sketches, having learned (though not explicitly) what parts of the world they refer to, which pieces they disregard, just exactly how they simplify" (1993: 176). Jordan questioned the underlying premise that teaching and learning should rely on visualism in the first place. It is worth noting that the childbirth educators whose classes I observed in fact devoted time to physical activities and bodily engagement. One instructor, a doula and former midwife, held a women-only class during which pregnant women crouched on their hands and knees in a pose that she and other midwives recommended for relief of back pain, and straddled exercise balls in postures for labor, and sank into squats to practice positions for pushing.

The physicality of the class contrasted with the visuality emphasized in all of the birthing classes I observed. In all five programs, visualization techniques were taught as a method of self-management during labor. "Visual imagery is a journey of the mind to a relaxing place," suggests *Prepared Childbirth the Family Way*, a booklet distributed at the hospital-based Lamaze classes that I observed. "Its purpose is to reduce tension by concentration on a mood and a place apart from your present situation" (Amis and Green 2002: 23). An exercise in the book, *Hypnobirthing: A Celebration of Life*, involved relaxing different parts of the body while imagining (both visualizing and reciting) letters of the alphabet as practice for managing labor. One instructor led the women in her class through an exercise that involved imagining the cervix "ripening, opening and blooming like a flower." An information sheet titled "Turning a Breech Baby to Vertex" counseled pregnant women to "enlist your mental powers to help turn the baby" and "silently picture what you want to happen."

Martin (1992[1987]) described and discussed the significance of metaphors and images of production and work in the lived experiences of reproduction in the United States today. Early medical literature portrayed human bodies as machines that worked in an orderly and predictable manner, and women's bodies in particular as flawed versions of men's bodies. In the early twentieth century, the anatomy and physiology of pregnancy and parturition were described in analogies with factories and assembly lines. Babies became products, and doctors themselves the managers or the skilled workers who delivered them. Women were workers or, alternatively, they were machines, which over the course of the twentieth century replaced skilled laborers. Martin suggested a relationship between these images and metaphors and the obstetric practices now considered standard in hospitals. A direct line of communication between the baby and the doctor is established by fetal monitoring, the use of which is now in question.[6] In successive versions of *Williams Obstetrics,* a textbook that is used by generations of doctors in scores of medical schools, Martin noted changes in the description of labor that literally write the woman out of the picture. While the tenth edition, published in 1950, described labor as "the series of processes by which the mature, or almost mature, products of conception are expelled from the mother's body," the sixteenth edition, published in 1980, includes no mention of the mother or her body, except in reference to "intra-abdominal pressure" (Martin 1992[1987]: 147). "There is a compelling need for new key metaphors, core symbols of birth that capture what we do not want to lose about birth" (1992: 157).

Childbirth educators echoed these sentiments. They chose carefully the metaphors and images that were presented in birthing classes, recognizing their significance as the cultural and social resources from which American middle-class women and men draw as they experience childbirth. Instructors drew attention to the choice of words that describe birth, insisting that a healthy woman in labor is not a "patient" because pregnancy and parturition are not diseases. Klassen, in a study of home birthing women in the United States, suggests, "Their subtle shifting of the language of birth reflects these convictions about birthing, as they replace the conventional phrase 'to give birth' with the more active 'to birth'" (2001: 5). When Carol, a doula and former midwife, talked in her classes about risk, she was describing the possibility of negative effects from medical interventions in the hospital. Privately, she also told me that she considered home, not hospital, a safe space for birth—inverting the logic that most American middle-class women and men take as given. Childbirth educators also were concerned with acknowledging sensuality and sexuality as part of the experience of pregnancy and birth. Physical exercises practiced in the classes typically involved pregnant women being held and supported by their partners, who were taught massage techniques that could be applied as comfort measures in labor. Pregnant women and their partners were also advised on the relationship between a woman's sexual arousal and the stimulation of labor. Physical intimacy, childbirth educators told them, contributed to natural childbirth.

Childbirth educators were concerned especially with countering birth "horror" stories that emphasize pain, suffering, complications, and problems of childbirth. "Most women in North American now gain their first ideas of birth from television portrayals of birth in hospital dramas or sitcoms," midwife Ina May Gaskin observes. "Commercial television feeds on the sensational and the danger-charged moment" (2003: 164). In popular culture, childbirth is portrayed as an emergency—such as on medical reality shows like "Maternity Ward"—or as a comedy with water breaking unexpectedly and women screaming uncontrollably. In response, one childbirth educator showed her classes the opening sequence of the 1983 film, "Monty Python's The Meaning of Life," which portrays a normal hospital birth. Filmed from the perspective of the birthing woman, the sequence is intended as satire, featuring attendants who rush and bumble the woman on a gurney to the delivery room (then leave her in the hallway) and a pompous doctor who demands "the machine that goes 'bing'" be brought into the room. The sequence ends with the woman futilely calling, "Is it a boy or a girl?" after the mass has exited with her baby.

During the class, the sequence drew laughs, but during the discussion that followed, expectant parents expressed their feeling that the satire was thinly veiled. Kerri later described to me her experience of Cesarean delivery in terms of the film. Kerri had been in labor from 1 in the morning until noon that day, then pushing for more than three hours. "They say when you're in that pushing stage, the uterus should be doing 70 percent of the work and you're only doing

30 percent," Kerri recalled, "but I think it was probably reversed."
Exerting herself, she said, "I actually broke a lot of the blood vessels
in my eyes." As her contractions began to slow, the nurse-midwives
became concerned for her and her baby, and asked an obstetrician
to examine Kerri. He recommended a Cesarean section. "It was an
incredible transition because the minute we said, 'OK, do it,' it was
like this flood of people in the room, and the whole atmosphere
in the room, which had been one of patience and waiting and observing the natural process—everything changed," she said. As she
was taken on a gurney to the operating room, Kerri recalled, "I said
something—'This is just like the Monty Python movie'—and I don't
know. Nobody laughed. They didn't get the reference."

Kerri's story demonstrates the significance of literacy in ordinary
pregnancy. Whether they involve reading traditional print media
or writing in new forms of text (like apps)—or even a Monty Python movie recalled in the middle of birthing a baby—literacy practices influence and shape the everyday experiences of pregnancy
and childbirth for American middle-class women. Feminist scholars
have contended that texts such as pregnancy books and birthing
classes have been important tools for the policing and social control
of women. Yet, as I have demonstrated here, women themselves are
critical of the texts, strategically consulting a range of sources and
"shopping around" for the information and advice that they want
and need. Indeed, the intersections of literacy and consumption—
both ordinary practices of pregnancy and parenting in the United
States—will be examined further in later chapters of the book.
Women in my study looked to books and other texts as resources to
make sense and meaning of their pregnancies. For American middle-class women, pregnancy is a literacy event.

Notes

1. Armstrong, in her account of fetal alcohol syndrome (FAS), notes that
   the risk of FAS has become universalized so that "according to the official
   prohibitions of the US surgeon general, *all* pregnant women who drink
   are at risk of having a baby with fetal alcohol syndrome" (2003: 218).
2. "Parenting today is virtually synonymous with worry" (Apple 2006: 1).
3. A recent survey of pregnant women and new mothers found that only
   14 percent of respondents had experienced "natural childbirth," which
   makes it far from average and ordinary (DeClerq et al. 2006).
4. However, Carine M. Mardorossian (2003), in her analysis of Bradley
   classes, reaches conclusions similar to Armstrong (2000). Mardorossian

suggests that although the Lamaze and Bradley methods are perceived to be vastly different, they both seem to serve the interests of hospitals, not women and their partners.

5. Childbirth education classes were designed for married heterosexual couples, as book titles like Robert Bradley's *Husband-Coached Childbirth* (the basis of the Bradley method) suggest.

6. In 2009, the American College of Obstetricians and Gynecologists revised its guidelines on the use of electronic fetal monitoring during labor (Brody 2009). Yet, the American discourse on reproduction still tends to reduce pregnancy and childbirth to biology and to maintain a focus on babies and fetuses.

Chapter 2

PROTOCONVERSATIONS OF THE HEART
BELLY TALK

> The times that I get the most emotional are when I think about
> communicating with whatever it is inside. I think maybe that's
> when I imagine it as a baby—a future baby. Because I can translate
> from whatever that experience is to talking to an actual baby.
> —Dana at nineteen weeks pregnant

At nineteen weeks pregnant, Dana had received the results from her amniocentesis, which were "negative" or normal. She also learned that she was expecting a girl. Friends and neighbors already were offering their congratulations as well as their help and hand-me-downs for the baby. Dana was especially grateful for the offers of help, like making meals or babysitting, because she would have this child on her own. She was thirty-six years old, established in her career as an obstetrician, single, and ready to have a child. She became pregnant after six cycles using donor insemination. She had chosen the donor in part because he was a graduate student in music and Dana, an accomplished pianist and singer, liked this connection. Dana felt healthy and happy, but she also felt hesitant about the "fuss" that friends and neighbors were making. "It's still not like a baby to me yet," she explained. "It's a little thing inside, that's all. I don't think of it as human." Instead, she described "it" as a "pea" or a "bean" or a "peanut." Yet, when I later asked if she ever talked to her belly, Dana admitted, "I do, actually. Yeah, I do. Oh, I'll probably get all teary." After a pause, she continued, "Obviously—I don't know why—I get so emotional about it. Like, last night, she was— and also, when I transition from 'it' to 'she' consistently, that will be

very interesting for me, too. Usually, I feel a lot of movement starting around three or four in the afternoon, but last night, it was like
really, really active while I was trying to go to sleep. So, it was like,
'Wow, you're really busy in there.'"

Dana's story calls attention to the significance of language in the
making of a baby. Talking, reading aloud, and singing to the belly
were activities that frequently were described to me, and that I occasionally observed, during my fieldwork. Playing music, which
referred typically to listening to recordings or the radio (not performing it), also figured significantly, as did touching, patting, and
massaging a pregnant woman's belly. Such activities, which I call
"belly talk," were prescribed widely by experts and advice mongers
as prenatal stimulation or even prenatal learning.

In this chapter, I examine belly talk as a practice of ordinary pregnancy in the United States today. My aim here is not to evaluate
the claims made about belly talk in terms of child development, but
to examine their cultural significance. The importance ascribed to
belly talk illustrates American middle-class ideologies of language,
or ideas about what language is and what it does. It also illuminates
American middle-class expectations about babies, mothers and fathers, families and kinship, and persons. Dana and other pregnant
women and men in my study described belly talk as meaningful experiences. One woman whom I met during fieldwork said that she
and her husband had started to talk and read children's books to her
belly almost as soon as they saw the results of her home pregnancy
test. Other women described talking to the belly as they began to
feel movement. As the faintest flutters became more perceptible
as rolls, punches, and kicks, pregnant women described a growing
sense of something, if not someone, else being present. "It's just
very cool to think about a little thing inside and what it might be,"
Dana confessed. Talking to the belly involves and invokes meaningful acts of imagination. Dana did not talk to the belly because "it"
was a person already. Rather, talking to it was part of how the "little
thing inside" becomes a baby—and how Dana and other women
and men, relating to it, came to be mothers and fathers (Han 2009b,
2009c). For American middle-class women and men, belly talk is an
ordinary practice of pregnancy through which babies and mothers
and fathers become imagined and embodied.

I use the term *belly talk* in order to draw attention to the fact that
this is a communicative practice involving a pregnant woman and a
child that is imagined or expected. What is observed in everyday life
is a pregnant woman (or her partner or another person) talking to

her *belly*. I use the term also to reference scholarship on "baby talk," which also has been called "motherese" and refers to what linguists describe as a register (or verbal style) of language that American mothers, among others, use with children (Ferguson 1977). However, my use of the term is *not* intended to imply that belly talk is a form of baby talk. In standard American English, baby talk has been characterized as a "simplified" register (or verbal style), as exhibited in shorter sentences and Baby Talk words ("tummy" versus stomach) (Ochs and Schieffelin 1984). I did not find that pregnant women necessarily use the baby talk register with their bellies. Baby talk also has been thought to be a tool for language acquisition and more specifically for caregivers teaching language to children. However, this has been refuted in linguistic anthropology, where attention has turned from a narrow focus on baby talk to a broader concern with the processes of language socialization (Kulick and Schieffelin 2004). In this chapter, I argue that belly talk is the language socialization of pregnant women as mothers.

Cultural Expectations

At thirty-two weeks pregnant, Betsy laughed when I asked her if she ever talked to her belly. "You know," she said, resting her hands on her belly, "a lot of people ask me, 'Do you talk to the baby? Do you read?'" It seemed to Betsy that everybody knows today that talking to the belly, like eating right and exercising regularly, is part of the prescription for an ideal pregnancy. Pregnancy books, magazines, and Web sites—not to mention well-meaning family members, friends, neighbors, and strangers at the supermarket—advise pregnant women and their partners to talk, sing, and read aloud to the belly. On television programs and in feature films, pregnant women and other characters are depicted engaging in belly talk, both to stimulate a baby's development and to establish attachments and bonds.

However, Greta expressed surprise that this topic might interest me as an anthropologist. First, she suggested that belly talk seemed too trivial and unremarkable to study. Then she clarified that *her* belly talk was nothing out of the ordinary and as a result not worth documenting. "I haven't really done anything in particular," she explained, almost apologetically. "I sort of talk to her. I say, 'Hi,' and stuff, but I don't really get into conversations." Although most of the sixteen women with whom I recorded interviews described talk with their bellies, it is unclear how common it is and how long it has been practiced in the United States. The attention given to belly talk, not only in advice literature, but also in popular culture, suggests it is an ordinary practice of pregnancy in the United States today. Yet, from the perspective of history and anthropology, it is rather unusual. In an informal, and by no means exhaustive survey of American pregnancy books from the 1940s onward, I found no references to practices involving talking to the belly until the 1980s. Although I did not undertake a systematic study with grandparents, few of that generation whom I met during fieldwork recalled engaging in belly talk as pregnant women and expectant parents themselves.

When pregnant women and other adults or children talk to the belly, they ostensibly connect and communicate with whoever or whatever it is inside a woman's body, and as Morgan reminds us, "The social recognition of fetuses, newborns, and young children is embedded within a wider social context" (2006[1990]: 30). In contexts where the status of a pregnancy, fetus, or infant is considered uncertain—and human language is considered appropriate and relevant for humans only—belly talk, as an everyday experience, is unlikely to make sense. Morgan (1997) tells us that pregnant women in the Ecuadorean highlands talk about not fetuses or babies, but *criaturas*. In the village in Papua New Guinea where linguistic anthropologist Don Kulick (1992) conducted fieldwork, unborn children were not regarded as human and were referred to as "the belly." After they were born, infants might be talked about, but seldom talked to, as they were considered to lack human sense or understanding. Ochs and Schieffelin noted that Samoan infants from birth until the age of five or six months were called *pepemeamea*, translated as "baby thing thing" (1984: 295). Although talked about and occasionally talked to, mostly in the form of song or rhythm, infants in Samoa, too, were not treated as conversational partners—in contrast to the chat and chatter surrounding not only newborn infants, but also pregnant bellies and imagined or expected children in the United States.

Ivry (2010), in her ethnographic account of pregnancy in Japan, tells us that there is a long tradition of *taikyo* or "fetal education," that encourages pregnant women talk to their unborn babies. She reminds us that *taikyo* must be understood "as part of a broader understanding of the baby as a living being within an interconnected social environment" (Ivry 2010:153), which is both particular to Japan and predates the development of technologies such as the sonogram. Especially significant also is that the talk Ivry describes is not framed as a conversational "exchange" between pregnant woman or mother and imagined child, which is a critical feature of the belly talk that I consider here. Language researchers have referred to this type of exchange as *protoconversation,* which I reference in the title of this chapter. In contrast with an actual conversation that involves exchanges between two or more participants, in a protoconversation, a mother assumes the child's role in addition to her own. She interprets the child's actions, facial expressions, or vocalizations. She adopts what she imagines as the child's perspective, giving voice to the child's ideas or intentions.

Compared with caregivers in other societies, Ochs and Schieffelin (1984) have noted, white middle-class American mothers (along with English, Scottish, Australian, and Dutch mothers) typically engage even very young infants in protoconversations, and American mothers especially are oriented toward accommodating children. This can be seen materially in "baby clothes, baby food, miniaturization of furniture, and toys" and behaviorally in "putting the baby in a quiet place to facilitate and ensure proper sleep; 'baby-proofing' a house as a child becomes increasingly mobile, yet not aware of, or able to control, the consequences of his or her own behavior" (Ochs and Schieffelin 1984: 286). Linguistically, Ochs and Schieffelin observed among American middle-class mothers "the willingness of many caregivers to interpret unintelligible or partially intelligible utterances of young children" (1984: 288).

Belly talk emerges in a social context where pregnancy can be taken for granted as known fact, the survival of children is normal, and adult attachment and accommodation to even very young infants is seen as only natural. It arises also out of the conventional wisdom that stimulation—in the form of talk and toys—is necessary for the normal and natural development of a child.[1] In fact, the importance of stimulation is not a notion shared across all cultures and societies, which all have their own "ethnotheories" of child rearing and child development (Harkness and Super 1996). Anthropologist Meredith Small (1998) explains that Dutch parenting emphasizes the importance of regularity, rest, and cleanliness.

In the United States, expert advice to pregnant women and product advertisements in pregnancy magazines both promote talking to the belly as the stimulation needed for an imagined child's intellectual, emotional, and social capacities—that is, learning and bonding. While the author of *Pregnancy and Childbirth,* a popular pregnancy guide, gently suggests that expectant parents should "feel free" to interact with an expected child—reassuring readers not to worry about "depriving" the child if they "don't feel comfortable" with belly talk (Hotchner 1997: 42)—other experts and advice mongers emphasize the life-long influence of so-called prenatal stimulation or prenatal learning. William Sears and Martha Sears, the husband-wife, doctor-nurse authors of a popular series of books on pregnancy and infant and child care, tell their readers: "Orchestra conductors have claimed they feel an unexplained familiarity with music their mothers played while pregnant" (Sears and Sears 1997: 224).

In an article titled, "What's Going on in Your Baby's Mind?" *Baby Talk*, a parenting magazine distributed for free in the offices of obstetricians and pediatricians, explains to its readers: "The learning starts with the sounds and sensations a baby experiences before he's even born" (Henry 2001: 48). The same issue carried an advertisement for a product that allowed expectant parents to hear and record "sounds in the womb," such as "heartbeat, kicks, and hiccups," and also to broadcast their talking, singing, and playing music into the uterus. It described the product as "Brain Food for Your Baby (before your baby is born)." In another pregnancy magazine, an advertisement for a program called BabyPlus promises a "prenatal curriculum" of "audio lessons" that produce "improved school readiness and intellectual abilities" as well as "longer attention spans." The advertisement tells readers: "You're never too young to learn. (In fact, you don't even have to be born!)"

While I admit to harboring reservations about the claims made for prenatal stimulation and prenatal learning, my aim here is not to appraise them, but to consider the appeal they might have. First, it ought to be noted that the makers and marketers of products like BabyPlus make mention of "studies" in their advertisements. One of the most frequently cited studies is a paper by psychologists Anthony De Casper and Melanie Spence (1986) on what they called the prenatal experience hypothesis. While the study is cited as evidence of the effectiveness of teaching and learning even in utero, De Casper and Spence were testing the hypothesis that an infant's preference for his or her mother's voice after birth might be linked to exposure to maternal speech during the last six weeks of pregnancy. In their study, the psychologists found it was.[2] However, they did not draw conclusions about the educability of the baby in the belly. The references to "studies" in both the advice literature and in advertisements seem intended to give the impression that science backs their claims about the importance and necessity of talk to the belly.

Second, the idea that "you're never too young to learn" speaks directly to the cultural logic of middle-class Americans, whose belief in school, work, and family and their faith in mobility are rooted in assumptions about language, especially what it is and what it does. Birds sing, bees dance, and all kinds of animals can communicate, but human language is supposed to be uniquely complex and diverse. Literacy long has been supposed to distinguish the "progress" of human societies (Street and Besnier 2009[1994]). Within a given society, learning to talk and then especially to read and write are regarded as milestones in a child's development into a person, that is, an able, mature, full member of that community (Kulick and Schieffelin 2004). In the United States, and especially for white middle-class Americans, having ability in the uses of language, especially literacy, is seen as essential for success in school and work (Baquedano-Lopez 2004; Heath 2001[1984]; Long 2003).

Developing such abilities from an early age—apparently even in utero—is recognized as an advantage. This is especially salient in the face of the "fear of falling" that Barbara Ehrenreich (1989) has observed so haunts middle-class Americans in the late twentieth and now early twenty-first century. "Success" in life—that is, membership in the middle class—is seen as success in work, which depends on school. In turn, success in school depends on home, family, and parents in particular. Educators today regard parental involvement as a factor in student achievement. Beginning even in preschool, teachers cultivate involvement by imposing "backpack checks" that require parents to read and sometimes sign and return children's homework and other notices sent home from school. During pregnancy, advice on the development of attachments and bonds emphasizes the apparent need to start not just soon, but sooner. On the one hand, the authors of *What to Expect When You're Expecting* remind readers, "It's much more important for a baby to be taught that he or she is loved and wanted than to be taught how to speak and read"— and on the other hand, they advise pregnant women, "Any kind of prenatal communication may give you a head start on the long process of parent-baby bonding" (Eisenberg et al. 1996[1984]: 187).

The contradiction that is apparent in advice like this, in fact, reflects other tensions in the larger cultural and social context. American middle-class children today are both priceless and commodified. As sociologist Viviana Zelizer (1985) has observed, children are supposed to be subjects beyond the reach of markets—cared for, kept, and loved, not turned out to labor, circulated, or traded. "Properly loved children, regardless of social class, belonged in a domesticated, nonproductive world of lessons, games, and token money" (Zelizer 1985: 11). Ironically, the *devaluing* of children's ability and worth as economic producers led to their revaluation as "priceless." The withdrawal of children from the labor pool also led to the entry of American mothers into the work force in significant numbers during the early twentieth century (Zelizer 1985: 9). At the same time, the full-time "expert" mother—"well informed on scientific and medical matters pertaining to her family's health" (Apple 2006: 5)—became valorized.

At the turn of the twenty-first century, Hays (1996) observes that cultural contradictions mark an American mandate on what she calls intensive mothering. "In a society where over half of all mothers with young children are now working outside of the home, one might well wonder why our culture pressures women to dedicate so much of themselves to child rearing" (Hays 1996: x). Hays argues that the contradictions point to "a persistent, widespread, and irreducible cultural ambivalence about a social world based on the motive of individual gain, the impersonality of bureaucratic and market relations, and the calculative behavior of *homo economicus*" (Hays 1996: 154). However, others suggest that the logic of capitalism now largely informs child rearing. Historian Peter Stearns (2003) suggests that what was once the "wonderland" of childhood has become reimagined as the training ground for adulthood, with play reimagined as the "work" of children and parental attention regarded as "investment" into a child's future. Journalist Ann Hulbert (2003) notes how the metaphors of markets now frames popular ideas and practices surrounding children and parenting. "Popular experts, in addition to becoming public advocates, sounded more like management consultants to an on-the-go clientele as they peddled programmatic visions of child rearing in a high-tech, hectic era" (2003: 13).

The women whom I interviewed were wary, if not outright skeptical, of the new visions of high-tech and hectic parenting, and of the claims made for prenatal learning and prenatal stimulation. Rebecca had been collecting her favorite children's books. She and her husband read aloud Dr. Seuss's *One Fish, Two Fish, Red Fish, Blue Fish* to her belly one evening, but "just for fun," she explained. "I read somewhere that it's never too early to start reading to the baby—to expose it to different vocabulary," Bridget said. "But I'm like, who does these studies? How can they pick that up? For crying out loud, there's so much pressure once you're born." As a high school social studies teacher, Bridget herself felt that the early involvement of parents might instill in children the habits and interests that seem so vital to school and work. "I see so many kids that don't like reading," she explained, then quickly added, "But it could be that it's pushed on them." Greta, a high school special education teacher, poked fun at the kinds of activities that experts and advice mongers now promote to pregnant women. "I don't sit with headphones on my belly or do anything in particular. Nothing like book reading or going over times tables," she said, describing her own belly talk. "No flash cards yet—that'll come later," she joked.

In fact, Greta felt that the stimulation and learning activities prescribed to pregnant women in fact were "interfering" with the baby. In her opinion, a child required comfort and calm to develop and grow. "Sometimes I'll just lie down and I'll just put my hand on my stomach and I don't really say much or do anything," she said at twenty-eight weeks pregnant. "I just sort of lie there and think about her, think about what it's going to be like, or enjoy if I feel a kick. So, I guess that's what I've done for bonding—just a little quiet time to appreciate that I have life inside me and that she's growing. I'm housing her and nurturing her."

Although the women expressed skepticism about stimulation and learning in utero, they did not question the significance of language and literacy. Rebecca might have been reading to her belly "just for fun" and not for an instructional purpose, but her actions affirm literacy as "part of one's orientation to a lived reality made meaningful through the interpretation of text" (Baquedano-Lopez 2004: 246). Thus, in addition to reading pregnancy books and other texts, producing charts and records, and attending birthing classes (which I discussed in chapter 1), belly talk is one of the practices of pregnancy as a literacy event. I interpreted the skepticism that Rebecca and others expressed as an extension of their critical consumption of pregnancy advice. Rebecca, who held a master's degree, and Bridget and Greta, who both were high school teachers, themselves expert learners and teachers of language and literacy, easily could afford *not* to accept the information and advice that were proffered to them and still be responsible pregnant women and good mothers. In fact, given the especially close association between expert advice and product advertisement, rejecting the headphones and flash cards that Greta mentions can be read as appropriate parental consumption (which I discuss further in chapters 5 and 6).

Making a Baby

Language is supposed to distinguish humans from other animals. All kinds of animals can communicate, but people use language in ways that demonstrate still other capacities. They use language to make order and sense of their world—for example, to name and know each other. Nicole noted as significant when her husband, Joshua, began to refer to their child with the name that they planned to give her. Dana, whose story begins this chapter, chose her words with care. She called "it" not a baby, but "a little thing inside," and noted self-consciously that with the results of her amniocentesis, she has begun to refer to "it" as "she." Dana also insisted that she is not yet a mother. "I think of myself as a pregnant woman, which is describing me. You know what I'm saying? It's not describing my role that I'll have with respect to another person," she explained. "I don't know when I'll start to feel like a future mother, but not right at the moment. It's just very much about what's going on in my own body right now."

Dana did not think of "whatever it is inside" as yet a baby or of herself as yet a mother or a parent. At the same time, "it" mattered to her. Belly talk emerges in a context of liminality, or what Turner called a state of being "betwixt and between" that individuals occupy as they undergo rites of passage marking a change in their social status. Pregnancy has been described as a rite of passage, involving a pregnant woman's separation, transition, and incorporation from childless woman to mother. Pregnancy itself is liminality, and carries liminal feelings with it. A pregnancy can be both mistimed or unplanned *and* wanted, and a baby represents new roles and responsibilities that can be regarded with ambivalence. The pregnant woman is a liminal figure, no longer a childless woman, but not fully a mother. Liminal, too, is the baby in her belly, which is both human and not fully a person.

For Dana, admitting that she talked to "it" meant confessing that even at nineteen weeks gestation, "it" had become important and meaningful in powerful and human ways. Dana told me that this made her feel uncomfortable. As an obstetrician, she has been trained to look at pregnancy with a certain amount of detachment. Now, the pregnancy was *hers*. Dana also identified herself as a feminist committed to reproductive rights. She understood that her belly talk could be, in her view, misinterpreted. "I'm not sure in talking to it, I'm thinking of it as human necessarily," Dana explained, "because it's actually no different from the way that I talk to my pets." Although talk generally is recognized as what happens between people, it need not involve people only. People talk to other kinds of subjects and objects, like animals, plants, and machines, for various reasons and to varying effect. Dana talked to her cats. Though not people, her cats still matter to her. Talking to them demonstrates this, perhaps to her cats and perhaps to herself. Dana engages in play with her pets and expresses her affection for them.

People also talk to subjects whose presence can be questioned, notably in religious observance, where talk can be directed to a deity, spirits, or ancestors that cannot be seen, heard, or otherwise perceived. Webb Keane contends, "Language is one medium by which the presence and activity of beings that are otherwise unavailable to the senses can be made presupposable, even compelling, in ways that are publicly yet also subjectively available to people as members of social groups" (1997: 49). The real and present talk among real and present people stands for the realness and presence of the beings talked to and talked about. Talk to the belly makes the unseen, unknown, and uncertain "baby" in the belly real and present to the pregnant women, other adults, and children who engage it through talk.

At eighteen weeks, Bridget *knew* that she was pregnant, but she did not *feel* it. Morning sickness had affected her only mildly, making her a bit more tired after a day at work, teaching social studies at an area high school. Her home pregnancy test and her prenatal visits with the obstetrician told her that the pregnancy was a fact, but at eighteen weeks, there were no outward signs—her pants still fit her waist—and there were no inward signs. Bridget anxiously anticipated feeling fetal movements. She also looked forward to the sonogram that would be performed after twenty weeks because she and her husband could then see the baby, even learn its sex. "It's funny because sometimes—I don't forget that he or she is there, but it's just like, I don't feel it," she said. "So, I try to make a distinct effort to talk to him or her every day." For Bridget, engaging in belly talk was a way of feeling pregnant—that is, feeling that the baby she wanted was present with (or in) her.

"I read somewhere that by sixteen weeks, their hearing is [developing]," Bridget told me, "so as a mother, tell him or her stories or just talk to them because they can bond with your voice." Women and men in my study described as significant the ability of the child, even in utero, to recognize the voices of his or her mother and father. They emphasized it less in terms of learning and more in terms of bonding. Tim Ingold (2000) notes the importance and meaning that have been attached to the voice as revealing the "inner being" of a person.

> In speaking, the voice "sounds through" from the inside to the outside; in hearing it conversely penetrates from the outside to the inside. Where vision places us vis-à-vis one another, "face-to-face," leaving

each of us to construct an inner representation of the other's mental
state on the basis of our observation of outward appearance, voice
and hearing establish the possibility of genuine intersubjectivity, of
a participatory communion of the self and other through shared im-
mersion in the stream of sound. (2000: 246–47)

Sight and vision make available only "outward appearance." In contrast, the oral and the aural allow access to what is genuine. For
American middle-class women and men, belly talk offers the promise of the authentic, true, and real.

Making Parents

Women and men alike described the special significance of belly talk
as a means of making pregnancy real and present for men (Han
2009b, 2009c). Kris described the gap in understanding that existed
between her and her husband, David, during the first few months of
her pregnancy, before her belly had begun to swell. From her perspective, he did not and could not appreciate the range of impacts
that pregnancy made on her daily. Physically, she felt ill and fatigued.
Emotionally, she felt excited and overwhelmed. "It's like they get to
audit the class," remarked Kris, a graduate student. "They don't actually have to take the exam at the end." David admitted that he did
not think about the pregnancy as Kris did. Because he did not experience it in his body, he told her, it felt "unreal" to him.

Greta said that her husband, Adam, also seemed disconnected
from the pregnancy. Then came the twenty-week sonogram, when
they saw the baby and learned that they were expecting a girl, and
the first movements that Adam could feel, when he placed his hand
on Greta's belly. A flutter of activity followed. They picked out a
stroller, a paint color for the spare bedroom they planned to remake
as a nursery, and a name for the baby. They registered for classes on
childbirth preparation, breastfeeding, and infant care, enlisting in
weekend courses called "Basic Training for Moms" and "Boot Camp
for Dads." At twenty-three weeks pregnant, Greta took obvious
pleasure in Adam's stepped-up participation in the pregnancy and
his engagement with the baby. "Adam says, 'Hi,' and oh, you know,
'Give us a kick,'" she told me. "This morning, I could feel her move,
and she's been moving a lot, so I asked Adam to talk to her, and then
he did, so she'd kick. So, that's kind of fun."

Belly talk draws men into the experience of pregnancy, which
for David and Adam seemed unreal or disconnected from what they

could perceive. As a tactile experience, talking to the belly makes both belly and baby tangible. I arrived at this realization as I sat with Kevin and Betsy in their apartment one late afternoon. Betsy and I had been conversing about their plans for a home birth, which Kevin and Betsy had sought because they wanted both to be involved actively in the birth. "Men are totally taken out of it," Kevin had commented. "The world expects men to be smoking a cigar." The conversation drifted through Betsy's anticipation and anxiety about the birth. Then Kevin, seated on the floor at Betsy's feet, suddenly turned, pushed up the bottom of her shirt to expose her belly, and began to speak slowly and exaggeratedly into it. "Hello," he said, with his lips pressed near his wife's navel. "I love you."

Belly talk brings men into a close and involved relationship with the belly and the child imagined inside. "Last week, we saw the videos about birth. Somehow it helped me realize that what's in there"—Daniel gestured to his wife Martina's belly, burgeoning at thirty-three weeks—"is an actual person that's going to come out and I have to—that we have to relate to it and everything. Then I realized, well, I can start relating to the baby right now—talking to the baby while it's still in the womb." Popular pregnancy books, written for women, now include advice intended for men. "Your wife may have the edge in getting to know the baby prenatally because it's comfortably ensconced in her uterus, but that doesn't mean that you can't start to know the new family member, too," advise the authors of *What to Expect When You're Expecting,* in a special section of the book called "Fathers Are Expectant, Too" (Eisenberg et al. 1996[1984]: 413). "Talk, read, sing to your baby frequently," they suggest (413).

The making of a baby involves, significantly, the making of a parent or parents. When women and men in my study discussed their talking to the belly, they described engaging in role-play that appears to anticipate the roles that they will play as parents. I found especially striking the *gendering* of their roles. Susan Walzer has suggested that women and men become "channeled toward differentiation by social arrangements, and especially, by cultural imagery that constructs what it means to be a 'good' mother or father, wife or husband, woman or man" (1998: 7). In my study, women and men alike described men's belly talk as stories and games—for example, playing with the belly by poking or prodding it, even blowing raspberries on it, to prompt kicks and punches from inside the uterus. In contrast, women, like Greta, described their belly talk as comfort and calm.

For women, belly talk also has become a meaningful performance of kin work. Michaela Di Leonardo (1987) called attention to the

unrecognized work that women accomplish when they write holi-
day cards and letters and cook for family gatherings. She described
such activities as kin work, or "the conception, maintenance, and
ritual celebration of cross-household kin ties" (DiLeonardo 1987:
442). Not only do the responsibilities of kin work belong primarily
to women, but kin work also defines women as wives and mothers. Significantly, women's performance of kin work enables men to
stay connected to their family members and friends, such as when
wives keep abreast of the happenings of their in-laws and pass along
the news to husbands. Women's kin work includes creating situa-
tions that allow men to participate in family life, whether arranging
a birthday party or even passing the phone to have a husband say
hello to his mother.

Women perform kin work when they encourage men to engage
in belly talk. Martina told me that she had recruited her husband,
Daniel, to have a talk about a serious matter with their expected
child. At twenty-two weeks pregnant, Martina had been advised to
sleep on her side because lying on her back could cut off circulation
to the baby. She admitted that she had difficulty following this advice, and it worried her.

> Sometimes, I fall asleep on my back, and at some point in the middle
> of the night, I'll wake up. Oh my gosh, how long have I been on my
> back? This happened a couple of times. Finally, I said, "OK, Daniel, I
> need you to tell the kid something." So, he goes down, puts his head
> toward my stomach, and I told him to tell the baby that—who he was
> because it's not my voice, and it's a very deep voice compared to mine.
> You know, introduce yourself, and then say, "If you ever can't breathe
> or if Mommy is lying on her back, then kick Mommy really hard so
> that she can roll over, OK?" So, that was what we told the kid.

Interestingly, in the exchange that she describes, Martina has Daniel
introduce himself, based on his physical and relational distance from
the baby in the belly. It is due to Daniel's ability to talk to the belly
in close physical proximity, however, that Martina has him speak to
their expected child. Mother recruits father to talk with their child
about a serious matter.

As modern and new as belly talk appears to be, its gendered and
gendering uses seem familiar. Women and men become socialized,
through language, not as generic or gender-neutral "parents," but
as mothers and fathers. Ochs (1992) observed that ideas about gender become practiced in language, as when American middle-class
mothers not only interpret the utterances of their children, but also

voice for them. When a mother prompts her child to say "please" or "thank you," her own utterance is treated as if the child had spoken. "'Mother' is ignored because through her own language behavior, 'mother' has become invisible" (Ochs 1992: 355). Women repeat this pattern in belly talk as the language socialization of men as fathers. They acknowledged men's talk to the belly and underrated their own. Heather, thirty-two weeks pregnant, emphasized the significance of her husband Taro's belly talk. "Taro talks to the baby more than I do," she said. "The things I say to the baby are like, 'Oh, please don't kick me there.' They tend to be more like pleading with the discomfort than speaking with the baby." Betsy, then thirty-two weeks pregnant, said, "I talk to him or her a little bit. Kevin actually talks to him more than I do." The women in my study described men's belly talk with pleasure and pride. For women, it represented the kind of relationships that they had with their husbands as partners, and that they anticipated their children having with their fathers.

The Belly Talks Back

Women's expectations and experiences of their own belly talk encapsulate the complexities and contradictions of being pregnant. Pregnancy is physical and psychological, personal and political, private and public. The liminality of being pregnant comes from being betwixt and between not only childless woman and mother, but also one body and two bodies. In interviews, some women described their belly talk as having material effects on the body of the baby, prompting it to move and "exercise" or contributing to the development of its brain. Like food, talking to the belly provided sustenance to the child in utero. Women described belly talk as real and present, like a substance. They described even their thoughts as real and present communication with the baby in the belly. "I've read to him a couple of times, but it's more of an internal dialogue that I have than actually speaking—and I can believe that the baby can sense that," Betsy told me. "I don't know whether I'm right or not, but I think about him or her a lot and I'll talk to him, maybe not expressively or outwardly, but he's in my thoughts." With a smile, she added, "I haven't got any feedback yet from the baby other than kicks and stuff."

Considering pregnant women's thoughts as a form of talk to the belly prompts rethinking the distinctions made between unspoken, internal, private, mental thoughts and spoken, external, public, physical talk. The so-called mind/body dichotomy has been both taken for granted and challenged in contemporary American culture. In recent years, researchers have demonstrated the physiology of emotion, connecting laughter with the release of endorphins in the bloodstream, mapping areas of the brain that are involved in feelings of anger or sadness, and emphasizing a mind/body relationship. At twenty-four weeks pregnant, Nicole drew upon her training as a biologist to describe her communication and connection to the baby in her belly. "We know the baby can probably hear us now, though she or he doesn't seem to respond to anything," she said. "Sometimes, I'm sitting there thinking, 'OK, now, kick.' So, I'm trying to establish a psychic link: I tell the baby to kick and then *kick*." With her hand on her belly, Nicole flicked her finger to mimic the baby's response. "Because, you know, there's biology here. There are hormones," she explained. "But it doesn't work."

In addition to the belly talk of women and men, the belly's own talk figures importantly and meaningfully in the making of a baby. Pregnant women and other adults engaged in belly talk as a response to the belly's own talk or an attempt to provoke the belly to talk in the form of movement. Rolls, punches, and kicks were interpreted as expressions of contentment or discontentment and of preferences and opinions. The same movements, however, could give rise to different interpretations. A woman whom I met in a childbirth education class told me that her baby seemed to dislike loud rock music because it punched and kicked. Another women in the class, however, suggested that it was "just rocking out" or dancing to it.

"It's nice to have those moments when he's just going crazy in there," Betsy told me. "'Hi, what are you doing in there?' I just talk to him a little." For Betsy and for other women in my study, belly talk was an important act of imagination. Babies, persons, mothers and fathers, and families and kinship become imagined and embodied—in a word, made—through belly talk.

Notes

1. Recently, attention also has been drawn to the importance of gesture, to promote the development both of language and other abilities that language is supposed to support. "Don't just talk to your toddler—gesture, too," begins a news article circulated in newspapers and on the Web (Neergaard 2009). The article reports on the research of psychol-

ogists Susan Goldin-Meadow and Meredith Rowe, who examined the
language practices of parents and their possible effects on children. It
quotes Rowe, who says, "It wouldn't hurt to encourage parents to talk
more and gesture more." Previous studies had found that children from
low-income families started school with a more limited range of vocabulary than children from higher-income families. Because parents in
low-income families were observed using fewer words than parents in
higher-income families, parental speech has attracted concern. In the
new study, published in *Science,* Goldin-Meadow and Rowe documented
fewer gestures in addition to fewer words in low-income families.

2. De Casper and Spence suggested first that "newborns prefer their own
   mothers' voices, regardless of what she says, because of prenatal experience with her voice-specific cues" and second that "newborns will prefer
   the acoustic properties of a particular speech passage if their mothers re-
   peatedly recite that passage while they are pregnant" (1986: 134). After
   having pregnant women tape-record three passages, which they read
   aloud from story books, one group of women were asked to read aloud
   a target passage each day during the last six weeks of their pregnancies.
   Another group of women did not. Later, the infants born to the women
   in both groups were "tested"—while recordings of the three passages
   were played for each child, researchers recorded the number of sucks
   that he or she took on a pacifier. Based on previous studies, the infant's
   sucking pattern was taken as a measure of his or her preference, so that
   more frequent sucking was interpreted as a response to a familiar voice.
   De Casper and Spence found that infants whose mothers had read aloud
   daily preferred the recordings of their own mothers' voices reading the
   target passage, but also responded to unfamiliar voices reading the same
   passage. Infants in the target group showed no preference for the target
   passage. Based on their findings, De Casper and Spence concluded, "The
   fetuses had learned and remembered something about the acoustic cues
   which specified their target passage (e.g., prosodic cues such as syllabic
   beat, the voice-onset-time of consonants, the harmonic structure of sus-
   tained vowel sounds, and/or the temporal order of these sounds)" (1986:
   143).

Chapter 3

SEEING LIKE A FAMILY, LOOKING LIKE A BABY
FETAL ULTRASOUND IMAGING

J osie told me excitedly that she had some "cute baby pictures" to show me. "I wouldn't be a good mommy if I didn't," she exclaimed as she pulled them out from her wallet. When she handed me the thin, curling slips of paper, what I saw were grainy, white-on-black blurs that bore no resemblance to a baby. Josie, then four months pregnant, explained that they had been taken a few weeks earlier at a ten-week ultrasound scan, which her obstetrician had performed as a "quick look" for the heartbeat to confirm that she was pregnant. She then eagerly interpreted the pictures for me. "So, the baby was only about two inches. So, you can see—there's the probe here, and then there's the profile. There's the eye and the little nose. There's the big head, obviously, and the little body, and then his little legs fluttering out there," Josie explained. "I just say 'his,'" she added, because at the time, she did not know if she were expecting a boy or a girl. She slid the picture from the top to the bottom of the pile, directing my attention to the next image. As Josie narrated for me, a large, bulbous head and spindly, little arms and legs began to take shape, but try as I might, I still could not see as Josie did—as a "good mommy."

Carefully replacing the images in her wallet, next to photographs of family and friends, Josie told me that she and her husband now were looking forward to another scan at twenty weeks. This would be when the couple could learn the baby's sex, she explained. Josie planned to invite her parents and her grandmother to the screening as it presented an opportunity for the whole family to see the baby on the way. Later, when I met her after the second scan, Josie likened the experience to that of watching a movie together. "Amazing," she gushed. "It was like family bonding."

Josie's story illustrates the ways in which American middle-class women and men have embraced fetal ultrasound imaging or the sonogram as an ordinary technology. In interviews, when I asked pregnant women and their partners about their experiences with fetal ultrasound imaging, they typically mentioned the importance of "checking" on the baby and seeing that it was "OK," but also emphasized the scans were opportunities to see and "bond" with the baby, "find out" its sex or gender, and get its "picture." Not all of the partners in my study accompanied pregnant women on their prenatal visits with doctors or midwives, but none skipped the sonogram. Some, like Josie, viewed it as an event to invite other family members, especially grandparents and great-grandparents to-be. Scenes like the one that Josie described became familiar to me during the sonograms that I also observed during my fieldwork. Most scans I observed while I "shadowed" the staff at a clinic specializing in perinatal care. In addition, I observed scans while I accompanied interviewees on their appointments.

The fetal ultrasound scan is not only a routine of prenatal medical care, but more significantly, it has become a ritual of ordinary pregnancy. As such, it has provoked the interest of not only anthropologists and sociologists, but also art historians and legal scholars concerned with both the cultural contexts in which fetal ultrasound images become made and the social consequences that the uses of this technology have. I draw from their work in this chapter with the aim of introducing their insights to readers unfamiliar with both the practice of fetal ultrasound imaging and its scholarly critique. In particular, feminist scholars have been critical of the role of imaging technologies in the erosion of women's reproductive agency, arguing that the sonogram shifts authority from pregnant embodied women's experience to doctors' expertise and brings a change in focus from the pregnant woman to the fetus or baby (Petchesky 1987; Stabile 1992; Duden 1993; Dubow 2011). Indeed, ultrasound scans now figure into legal restrictions placed upon abortion services in the United States. The Guttmacher Institutes reports that as of July 1, 2012, twenty-one US states have written into their laws a requirement to offer or provide sonograms to any woman seeking abortion services, and another seven states require verbal counseling or written materials that inform women on accessing scans.

"The core and motivating belief is that a woman who sees her baby's image on a screen will be less likely to abort" (Sanger 2008: 358). Presented to women in terms of their "right to view," legal scholar Carol Sanger argues otherwise. "It is harassment masquerading as knowledge" (2008: 360).

Important and necessary as this perspective is, my aim is also to move beyond the current terms of discourse, not only on fetal ultrasound imaging particularly, but on pregnancy and reproduction more generally. Eugenia Georges has argued, "Although some feminist critics are certainly correct in pointing to the ways in which fetal imaging extends patriarchal medical authority over pregnancy, the strong demand for and enthusiastic reception of fetal imaging by pregnant women also suggests the emergence of a new consciousness, of their transformation into modern pregnant subjects" (1997: 105). This modern way of being pregnant in the United States is the focus of my study. In this book, I suggest a concept of the ordinary as a way to reorient studies in reproduction, which have been discussed primarily in terms of medicalization, technologization, and disruption.

In the previous two chapters, on literacy and on belly talk, I considered literacy and language as practices of ordinary pregnancy through which babies, parents, and families become made. In this chapter, I discuss what it is to see like a family, and how and why it is that the grainy white-on-black blurs look like a baby to pregnant women like Josie. I describe the taking of "baby pictures" at the sonogram as both the ritual and the record of the ritual. The scan is staged as a media and mediating event—a kind of Kodak moment involving baby pictures and family bonding. Building upon the broader understanding of literacy as a way of making sense and meaning of lived experienced through text, I suggest that the scan also might be understood as a literacy event. Pregnant women and others become taught how to "read" the images, which themselves are composed as baby pictures, following more familiar conventions in photography. The baby pictures then are incorporated, as texts and material objects, into other rituals of family and kinship, such as the keeping of a baby book or photography album and the sending of Christmas cards and birth announcements. Fetuses become imaged, and babies imagined, embodying the social relations and sentiments that we call family and kinship.

My analysis takes into account the context in which a baby picture is produced, circulated, and received in addition to the content and composition of the image itself. It is based in part on the approach that visual anthropologist Mary Bouquet (2000) has described. Bouquet suggests that an analysis of family photography can be illuminating for the study of kinship—not because it necessarily provides a record of family as it is, but because it is a practice *through which* family becomes imagined and embodied. In other words, the family photograph is a text through which the experience of family becomes lived. Bouquet observes that "family photography was and remains deeply involved in constituting kinship through the coherent looking images it produces, which are simultaneously material artifacts that occupy space and demand classification" (2000: 9). While fetal ultrasound imaging is not photography—indeed, the differences between the technologies is significant—its examination in terms of family photography illuminates the practices and ideas through which both baby picture and baby become made. Fetal images and (or as) family photographs are the texts of ordinary pregnancy and family life.

Routine and Ritual

Aside from the pregnancy test, fetal ultrasound imaging is one of the more widely used prenatal diagnostic technologies in the United States today. All but one of the pregnant women whom I interviewed had at least one scan performed. Only Betsy, who was preparing for a home birth, chose not to have a sonogram, which she could have had through her insurance. (The insurance did not pay for her home birth.) The decision had not been easy for Betsy to make and had been based on extensive reading and discussion with her midwives, who emphasized that the scans tended to cause more, not less, worry. In the end, Betsy reasoned that she had committed to a "nonmedicalized" birth and that she and her husband "will love this baby no matter what," which made the scan a moot issue for her. Still, she told me that she "felt tempted" by the thought of being able to see the baby's face.

Typically, women whom I interviewed had a scan performed between fifteen to twenty weeks, when they were advised to have a "level three" (detailed) sonogram in order to evaluate the condition of both the fetus and the organs that support the pregnancy, such as the placenta and cervix. Although doctors and midwives occasionally wheeled a portable imaging machine into a regular prenatal visit, the level three scan typically is performed by a sonographer at a specialized clinic. Based on what the obstetrician sees, the scan

might be the basis of a woman's decision to have other tests performed, such as an amniocentesis, which checks for genetic anoma-
lies that indicate conditions like Down syndrome.

In addition, scans also may be performed for a range of other reasons. When a pregnant woman has had irregular menstrual cycles
and cannot recall the dates of her last menstrual period, a scan is
used to measure fetal growth and calculate a due date. As with Josie,
a sonogram might be performed in a doctor's office during a prenatal visit as early as several weeks into the first trimester to detect a
fetal heartbeat and confirm a pregnancy. At other times, women
were referred to the perinatal clinic where I conducted fieldwork
to have a so-called viability scan. The staff at the clinic told me that
when they saw one on the schedule, they knew to be prepared for
a possible miscarriage. However, it was unclear to me whether the
women themselves understood this or even if the term "viability"
had been mentioned to them. While the clinic was known to be a
place where pregnant women with "risks" can seek care,[1] a number
of women told me that they were there simply because it had higher
quality equipment that would enable doctors to "see better."

The ability to see the growth and development of the fetus—
and to detect and diagnose problems with a pregnancy, including
its loss—has been touted widely as the benefit of fetal ultrasound
imagining. Being able to see the "baby" is experienced as a pivotal
moment for pregnant women. However, the feminist critique of the
sonogram is based on the recognition that seeing, like any other human activity, is as much conditioned by culture and society as by
biology—and that seeing itself *produces* the object that is being seen.
Lisa Mitchell (2001), in her ethnographic account of fetal ultrasound imaging in Canadian hospitals, describes how sonographers
do not simply show fetuses to pregnant women during their scans,
but narrate to them the significance of the black-and-white blurs on
the screen. Ostensibly, sonographers, with their expert eyes, merely
explicate the literal, objective reality presented during the scan. In
fact, fetal ultrasound imaging involves a kind of imagining (Han
2008, 2009a). Through the sonographer's show-and-tell, the blurs
become bodies and the bodies become ascribed with intentions and
emotions. What become produced during the scan are not only fetal
images and baby pictures, but fetuses and babies themselves. "The
fetal image is described, talked about, and sometimes talked *to* as if it
were an individual—and intentional, conscious, appealing, and sen-
tient person with meaningful ties to other people" (Mitchell 2001:
134).

Almost thirty years ago, feminist scholar Rosalind Petchesky (1987) cautioned that images of the fetus created powerful impressions because viewers believed that they were seeing literal, objective reality. Fetuses and babies become "real," with consequences for real women. On the one hand, there is the doctor who told me that her main concern was with women's health, and that she felt sonograms might help motivate some women to take their own care more seriously. A woman who might not quit smoking for her own health might do so for the sake of her child's well-being. On the other hand, this is now the exact same logic that is being used in some US states to require an ultrasound before an abortion. Whether the scans indeed motivate women to take (and seek) better care seems beside the point when we take into the account the manifold social determinants of health. The emphasis on medical and especially technological intervention, like the sonogram, deflects attention from the significant historical, political, and economic contexts and conditions in which women become pregnant.

In addition, the medical benefit of fetal ultrasound imaging is itself in question, with a number of medical researchers and practitioners cautioning that there is an overuse of the technology in the United States today. With the development of ever-more-sophisticated devices, there are expectations that the sonogram can be used to detect and diagnose a wider range of conditions, but evidence suggests that the expectations are outpacing the technologies themselves. Overall, studies show that the routine use of ultrasound scans has not necessarily improved the health and well-being of pregnant women, mothers, and babies.

For pregnant women themselves, the interest and even investment in fetal ultrasound imaging appears to have less to do with its medical efficacy than with its cultural and social experience. While it is a doctor's order that brings a woman into an ultrasound clinic, pregnant women bring their own expectations of the scan, regarding it as an opportunity to see the baby and take home its picture. Janelle Taylor (2008) describes the sonogram as a "hybrid" practice that straddles the needs and wants of biomedicine and of consumer society. She notes the tensions that can arise between clinic staff and pregnant women concerning the purpose of the scans. Increasingly, Taylor suggests, fetal ultrasound imaging has come to be associated with its entertainment value and treated as a consumer activity, as the establishment of so-called ultrasound boutiques underscores. In New York City, a boutique called A Peek in the Pod charged $295 for high-resolution prints, a CD-ROM of the images, and a DVD of the scan. Advertisements included disclaimers that the scans were not for medical, but for entertainment purposes (Santora 2004).

There were no ultrasound boutiques in the area where I conducted my fieldwork. The scans were marked as medical events in that they were performed during prenatal visits or at specialty clinics. Nevertheless, a number of pregnant women told me that they "had fun" at their scans. They were as likely to be interested in learning the baby's sex—in order to choose a name—as they were in "checking" on the condition of the pregnancy. Significantly, women also described the scans as enabling them to "go shopping" for clothing and other items in colors and designs regarded as appropriate for the child's gender, furthering the association between fetal ultrasound imaging and consumer activity. Insofar as the scans were understood to be medical events, women seemed to expect the confirmation of the healthy and normal condition of their pregnancies.

Still, not everyone experiences the scans as merely "checking" on the baby. For Kerri, whose reproductive history had included a miscarriage, a diagnosis of infertility, and two rounds of in vitro fertilization (both unsuccessful), the scans represented a "test" that she had to pass as a pregnant woman. "It felt like there were so many hoops that we had to jump through in the first trimester," she explained. "At any point, your joy could be shattered." In addition, the scans do not always offer the kind of confirmation that pregnant women in the United States today expect. The "viability" scan, which I described, is another case in point. Layne, whose work has examined American women's experience of pregnancy loss, observes that the use of technologies like fetal ultrasound imaging has effected "changing expectations regarding biomedicine's abilities to guarantee a live birth. Although women who have had a pregnancy loss are painfully aware that such events can occur, and experience and respond to subsequent obstetrical care and technologies differently as a result, most women at the beginning of their childbearing careers are ignorant of how common pregnancy losses are" (2003: 93). Layne comments on how adept women themselves become at reading the images, recognizing problems on the screen during a scan.

Elizabeth Peel (2009) found that more than one third of the respondents in her study on lesbian and bisexual women's experiences of pregnancy loss had suffered what she calls silent miscarriage—one that is discovered through ultrasound or other clinical intervention. Peel contends the loss is especially devastating ("It was a total shock") in part because women today approach fetal ultrasound imaging with excitement and even confidence ("We had no idea"), not fear (2009: 725). My own personal experience echoes her finding. Not long after I had begun my fieldwork, I took a home pregnancy test that confirmed the news. At about twelve weeks, during my first prenatal visit, my husband and I listened eagerly for a heart-beat as the CNM moved a Doppler device around my belly. After a pause, she apologized for the trouble, and said she would bring in a scanner, which at this early stage of pregnancy meant a vaginal ul-trasound. My husband and I peered hopefully into the screen while the CNM pointed out my uterus and then the small gestational sac. It was empty. Later, my husband said he had thought at first that the machine itself must have been defective because what a sonogram is supposed to do is show the baby. "The gap between faith in technol-ogy and the harsh reality of pregnancy loss seems especially great for men" (Layne 2003: 95).

A Kind of Kodak Moment

The ceiling-to-floor curtains whisked closed behind me. Gradually, my eyes adjusted to the dimness of the room. I was on time for my appointment to join Amanda and Phil at their twenty-week scan, but the sonographer was running ahead of schedule, and they were so eager for the sonogram. Amanda, lying on an exam table, smiled and nodded to me, then moved her eyes back to a monitor that had been angled for her to view. Her husband, Phil, hovered at her side, fascinated not only with the images of their baby, but also with the technology that produced them. His attention shifted between the monitor that Amanda viewed, and the one that the sonogra-pher used. Amanda had pulled up her shirt right under her ribs and pulled down her pants just around her hips so that her belly was exposed. With a gloved hand, the sonographer ran a device called a transducer across its surface, which had been lubricated with a layer of blue silicone gel. For the entire forty minutes of the scan, all eyes stayed on the bright white images flickering on the screens.

For Amanda and other pregnant women in my study, to see the baby at the sonogram was to believe that it was present in the belly. "It was like reality," Josie explained. "It wasn't really real until we saw it." As with belly talk, fetal ultrasound imaging makes the baby available to the senses. Talking to the belly makes the unseen, un-known, and uncertain baby real and present to the speakers who engage it through talk that is real and present. At a sonogram, one can see the images of the baby as they flash on the television screen or computer monitor, and one can touch the slips of paper onto which the images have been printed. The material reality of the paper is equated with the "realness" of the baby, as Layne (2003) notes in her study of pregnancy loss in America. "Sonogram photos and scraps from fetal monitors are frequently saved by bereaved parents and utilized as evidence to prove to others that a 'baby' existed" (Layne 2003: 97).

The image itself is regarded as not only a confirmation for the viewer, but also recognized as "literally an emanation of the referent," as French cultural critic Roland Barthes described the significance of photography (Barthes 1980: 80). "From a real body, which was there, proceed radiations which ultimately touch me, who am here; the duration of the transmission is insignificant; the photograph of the missing being, as Sontag says, will touch me like the delayed rays of a star," he writes, applying physics to the poetics of photography. "A sort of umbilical cord links the body of the photographed thing to my gaze: light, though impalpable, is here a carnal medium, a skin I share with anyone who has been photographed (1980: 80–81). Photography, as Barthes describes, is an embodied experience. By describing photography in terms of an umbilical cord—which is iconic of the connection between mother and child—Barthes suggests that taking a picture or having one's own picture taken, and seeing or showing it, are themselves a kind of kin making.

The fetal ultrasound scan has come to be a rite of passage for pregnant women in the United States. First, it involved seeing the baby as "real." Second, because most of the women in my study were scheduled to have an ultrasound scan performed at twenty weeks, it marked a halfway point in the forty weeks of pregnancy. Third, it also coincided with two other significant milestones that mark American pregnancy. By twenty weeks, women described their pregnancies as "showing," and that they were now "telling" the news of their pregnancies. They also described feeling movement inside the uterus.

Davis-Floyd (1992) noted that if pregnancy is a rite of passage, then showing and especially telling are part of the transformation of women—into pregnant women and expectant mothers—in the public domain. Several women had told me that they had continued to wear their regular, prepregnancy clothing until the fifth month. (For women who previously have had children, showing usually occurs earlier in the pregnancy.) Now that their pregnancies could no longer be concealed, they shared their news with neighbors, friends, co-workers, and others to whom they had chosen not to disclose their pregnancies, for various reasons. For some women in my study, receiving medical reassurances contributed directly to their decision finally to tell. Pregnant women were concerned especially with how the news might be received at work. A sign of their status as educated middle-class professionals, they generally were worried less about unfair treatment and more about unwanted attention. One pregnant woman whom I knew had decided not to discuss her pregnancy until well into her second trimester, in contrast with a co-worker who had announced it "practically from day one." "That was all anybody would talk about to her," she recalled. "It also just seemed like she was pregnant forever." Although Rebecca had shared the news with immediate family and close friends, she told me that she was reluctant to do so at work because she thought it would be "distracting." She did not want the attention drawn to her pregnancy, or the constant stream of questions (how she was feeling, when the baby was due) from well-intentioned colleagues.

In addition to showing and telling the pregnancy, the twenty-week scan also coincided with pregnant women's first experiences with feeling movement inside the uterus. This moment traditionally has been known as "quickening," and historically, it was the point at which a woman became regarded (and regarded herself) as pregnant. Most American middle-class women today no longer rely upon the bodily sensations of quickening. In fact, as feminist scholars comment, women might not necessarily even trust their feelings of movements. Some women in my study described not recognizing movement until after the twenty-week scan, which made seeing the kicks and punches onscreen all the more enjoyable. One woman told me that seeing the baby spin and stretch at the scan helped her "make sense" of the flutters and taps that she felt in her body.

Tracing the history of visual representations of the unborn from the eighteenth century to the present, Duden contends, "Motherhood, pregnancy, and birth are no longer somatic experiences of women expecting a child that will come, but the result of acceptance and interiorization of biomedical measurements" (1999: 24). Indeed, women in my study relied upon medical diagnostic technologies, such as the home pregnancy test and fetal ultrasound imaging, for confirmation of and information about their pregnancies. As Rebecca recalled of her scan:

> I had read that even with encephalitis, the baby could still be kicking, so it wasn't even reassuring to me that the baby was kicking. We

could go in there, and find out this awful thing. Of course, it turned out fine. [Laughter.] That's when I really started getting comfortable with telling people. To see that, OK, there are four chambers of the heart. There are the two kidneys. They're measuring the femur. The baby doesn't have a cleft lip. It was a detail in a way that just was extremely reassuring—because really by then, most things are formed.

With her master's degree in public health and career as an analyst for a research company, Rebecca herself would admit to have accepted and interiorized the importance of biomedical measurements and statistical probabilities. In fact, she had prefaced her recollection of the scan by telling me that she had read "too much" about pregnancy, and specifically about potential problems with a pregnancy. For Rebecca, the medical "views" of the vital organs and various parts of the baby were as meaningful as any "cute" pictures that she received, or kicks that she felt.

Seeing the baby at the sonogram was especially significant for men, who also experienced it as a passage into expectant fatherhood. In a study that compared women's and men's experiences of fetal ultrasound imaging, Margarete Sandelowski noted "the effect of increasing the involvement of expectant fathers in pregnancy and, thus, has furthered a trend toward family-centered maternity care and a more egalitarian role for fathers that began in the 1950s" (1994: 231). For example, men were more likely to accompany their wives not only to the sonogram, but also to other prenatal visits, which now seemed "less gynecological or for women only" (1994: 236). Fetal ultrasound imaging provided opportunities to "make up for" the differences in what women felt and knew about the pregnancy and the men did not. The women and men in Sandelowski's study told her that the scan contributed to "not only the father-child bond, but also the marital relationship by bringing wives and husbands together" (1994: 236). The men whom I met in my fieldwork described the twenty-week scan as "amazing," "awesome," "cool," and "special." They said that they had been "choked up" and "emotional." "There is something really in there," one man remarked quietly as he reached for his wife's hand.

Nicole described a "big change" in her husband Joshua's attitude and behavior concerning the pregnancy. Two days before the scan, she told me, "I'm not really showing yet. I haven't felt movement up until this week. I'm hoping that when we have our big ultrasound next week that that will do a couple of things—reassure me that things are still going OK and also get my husband involved."

When I spoke with her two weeks later, Nicole happily described how "amazed" Joshua had been at the scan. He had taken to remarking on the baby's resemblance to Nicole's father. They had the same nose and chin, he claimed. Joshua also referred to the baby by the name that he and Nicole had chosen. They had learned that they were expecting a girl. They called her Carly.

The twenty-week sonogram itself presented an opportunity to pregnant women and other adults to bond with the baby through talk. At scans, I observed talk directed both to a woman's belly and to the images viewed onscreen. A woman touched her belly before her scan and said, "Showtime!" Another woman, seeing an arm move across the monitor, waved her hand and called, "Hi, baby." In general, there was little talk during the scans. Sonographers answered questions about what they were imaging—for example, pointing out parts of the body—but they made clear that the doctors were the experts on the "results" of the scans. After exchanging pleasantries before and after the sonograms, they otherwise maintained mostly silence as they performed the scans. Some couples and family members also remained silent during the scans. One woman explained to me that she had been "processing" the experience. Other couples and family members commented on the images, ranging from the resemblance of the child to its mother or father to the "alien" or "freaky" appearance of the fetus.

Women and men in my study experienced the medical technology of fetal ultrasound imaging in the terms of television, movies, and other familiar media. "We're lying there, and there's the monitor, and the lights go down, and then all of a sudden—I mean, it was a wonderful experience," Josie recalled of her ten-week sonogram. This was despite having to tolerate the discomfort of a scan performed with the transducer inserted into the vagina because the views of the uterus might be blocked by the pubic bone. Later, Josie also likened her twenty-week sonogram, to which her husband, her parents, and her parents-in-law had accompanied her, to watching a television show or movie together.

Megan had been advised that she could bring a blank videotape to her scan, and have it recorded. Her mother organized a family potluck to show the video. Siblings, cousins, aunts and uncles, and close friends from all sides of Megan's family attended the screening. After dinner, they settled around the TV. Megan's mother, the grandmother-to-be, passed around photocopies of a program that she had composed on her computer. It read:

The Stanley Production Company of Michigan Presents:
"The New 2003 Stanley Baby"
The First Preview: July 25, 2003
First Production: December of 2003

The first preview was the date of the family potluck, and the first production that of the due date. The program also identified Megan as "Production Stage Manager" and Megan's husband, Patrick, as the "Producer." Acting as master of ceremonies, Megan's mother opened an envelope that Megan handed to her. Displaying the flair of a presenter at the Academy Awards, she pulled out a card on which the sonographer had written the sex of the expected child. As she made the announcement—"It's a boy"—the gathering burst into talk, laughter, and applause. The audience immediately became hushed as the video began—even though no sound actually accompanied the scan.

Medical sonographers themselves recognized the significance of the sonogram's entertainment value. Joan, a sonographer whom I had shadowed, described an important part of her work to me as "giving a tour" or "putting on a show." Joan emphasized first and foremost the medical value of routine fetal ultrasound imaging. Over the years, she has developed her own way of working, literally from the head to toe of the fetus, to check off the boxes on her mental checklist of the views that the doctors required.[2] With

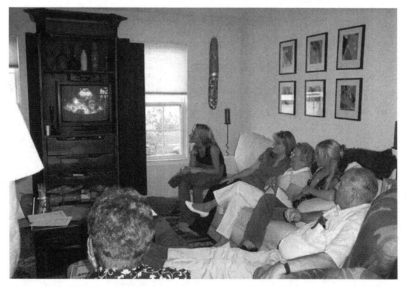

FIGURE 3.1. Family members gather for a screening of an ultrasound video.

one hand maneuvering the transducer across the pregnant woman's belly and the other pressing and clicking keys on her keyboard, Joan "froze" or captured images of the vital organs and labeled them. As she worked, however, she named the parts that flashed and pulsed on the monitors that she and the expectant parents viewed, giving a tour of the baby's body. From time to time, she also paused over a particular view or part, like the baby's face or hands or feet, putting on a show for the expectant parents. Sometimes, she stopped to print a picture.

Taylor (2004) comments on how the work of sonography, a paraprofession dominated by women, involves technical skills and skilled caring. Mitchell, in her study of fetal ultrasound imaging in Canadian hospitals, notes that doctors hired sonographers "not just for their technical skills, but also because they were 'friendly and know how to talk to patients'" (2001: 119). Both requirements were evident in the tours and shows that Joan gave (Han 2008). However, she also was well aware that her ability to capture the views required for prenatal diagnosis depended upon the cooperation of pregnant women. It is because they regarded the sonograms as enjoyable events that they tolerate the inconvenience and discomfort the scans might pose to them. The appointments, scheduled during office hours, meant having to take personal time in the middle of the workday and having to rearrange other responsibilities. At the clinic where Joan worked, women were instructed to drink water before they arrived as its presence in the bladder provided a medium for the sonar. I observed that women followed the instructions. They arrived early and waited patiently even with the discomfort that a full bladder poses to a woman who is five months pregnant. So, in fact, what Joan described as the "extras" and "little things" that she performed during the scan—like printing pictures for pregnant women to take home and recording the scan on a video tape—were also part of her job.

The shows and extras also enhanced Joan's own satisfaction, as a self-described people person, with her work. Although she maintained mostly silence as she performed the scans, and deferred medical questions to the doctors, Joan also answered questions about what kinds of views were captured during a sonogram and how the technology worked. From her perspective, the work of sonography also involved "educating" pregnant women and family members. This entailed sharing her own reading of the fetal images as texts, which pregnant women then shared almost word-for-word with family members and friends viewing the pictures, as I described in Josie's story above—and demonstrating for them an appropriate appreciation for the ability to read the texts and for the texts themselves. Thus, the sonogram can be read as itself a kind of literacy event. Literacy, as linguistic anthropologists have noted, refers to more than the ability to read and write. It encompasses a raft of ideas and practices that train individuals in particular moral sentiments, which also include the importance and meaning of reading and writing in everyday life. This is also a reason why Joan paid attention to both the medical and entertainment values associated with her work. An appreciation of the scan as "checking" on the baby and "bonding" with it *both* are feelings appropriate for pregnant women and expectant mothers and both are cultivated at the sonogram.

For American middle-class families, the twenty-week sonogram also is anticipated as the occasion when they can learn the sex or gender of the expected child. "That's the whole point of this," answered a grandmother-to-be, after Joan had asked the pregnant woman and her partner whether or not they wished to "find out" the sex of the baby. The reading of the fetal image as a text of sex and gender influences still other ideas and practices, notably concerning consumer activities. "Now I can go shopping," I heard on more than one occasion, not only from pregnant women, but also from their mothers and mothers-in-law as expectant grandmothers. At another scan, the pregnant woman and her partner were accompanied by both mothers, who were interested in knowing, as one of the grandmothers-to-be explained, "if it will be hockey skates or figure skates." The expectant father added hastily that it would be "hockey skates, either way." Presumably, he was demonstrating the value he placed on the imagined or expected child whatever its sex as well as correcting a gender stereotype that the older woman held (not to mention a personal preference for playing hockey over figure skating).

Sybil, whose daughter-in-law, Heather, was pregnant, had not been present at the ultrasound scan. Heather and Sybil's son, Taro, however, had brought home a video recording of the scan. "We saw the sonogram the other day. It's a video tape, and it's the first time I'd ever seen a video tape of a baby in utero. It's really, really exciting," Sybil told me. "I've only seen a photograph, you know, of a—what's it called? A scan? A sonogram. So, the little heart was beating—boom boom boom boom boom. Then the person circled the little eyes and the little mouth, and then it went down a beautiful, beautiful curve of the backbone all the way down to the tail—and they circled the little penis." Sybil laughed, then continued. "I told Taro and Heather that I didn't want to know [the expected child's sex], and didn't want them to tell me. They wanted to know. They definitely wanted to know, and were going to ask. But when they showed the whole [sonogram], you know, that's fine for me to know, too. Now they're planning the name and everything like that."

Learning the sex or "gender" of the expected child at the scan set into motion other rituals of kinship. "Planning the name" frequently became discussed as a reason why expectant parents were interested in determining if the expected child were a girl or boy. Heather and Taro planned to give their child, a boy, a Japanese middle name in celebration of his ancestry. Other couples also planned to give their children names that were meaningful within their families, and determining at twenty weeks whether they were expecting a girl or boy sometimes helped them to choose, especially when it upset expectations. From the time that she took her first pregnancy test, Amanda had been convinced from that she and her husband, Phil, were expecting a girl. In fact, they were planning to name their child after Phil's grandmother, whom Amanda, a self-described feminist, had admired as a woman "ahead of her times." Then, almost three months later, after the twenty-week scan, I received an e-mail from Amanda, with the subject line reading "It's a ..." In the first line of the e-mail came the announcement: "_BOY_!!!!!!!" The message continued: "Even I, as * sure * as I was that this was a girl, had to admit that the 'stem' we saw between those little legs looked convincing." With the news, Amanda's mother began "collecting"—that is, purchasing—clothes and toys for her expected grandson. Another couple, Elizabeth and Ethan, described a similar situation, though in their case, they learned at the twenty-week scan that they were expecting a girl. "I thought it was a boy before. I was picturing little overalls or suspenders—just, this little boy," Elizabeth confessed. "Then, when I found out it was a little girl, I thought, 'Oh, we can have tea parties!'"

The seeing and naming of body parts, especially of what Joan called "girl or boy parts," are significant in the making of a baby. At the fetal ultrasound scan, the baby becomes described and recognized in terms of its anatomy and physiology. It becomes biologized. It is no longer an abstract imagining or imaging of a baby, but a baby that has a body. The baby also becomes a text that is read aloud and interpreted for others. Certain parts are attached with special meaning, like the heart, with all its cultural (and medical) significance as a sign of life. At the sonograms, I observed pregnant women and other family members especially thrill to the sight of a baby's face, hands, and feet. Rebecca marveled over the two kidneys and the femur. Girl and boy parts marked the baby as natural and normal in that all human beings are supposed to be one or the other. Interestingly, what expectant parents saw at the sonogram was an indication of biological sex, but they preferred to talk about the baby's "gender." The talk of hockey skates versus figure skates and pictures of little overalls or suspenders supplanted by visions of tea parties all speak to the material significance of sex and gender in the making of a baby. The attention to body parts illustrates the importance and meaning of the body as materiality and the "realness" of the baby.

Baby Pictures

By introducing the idea of the ultrasound scan as a literacy event and the fetal images themselves as text, I also wish to emphasize the materiality of reading, writing, and the text themselves, which I discuss here. Fetal ultrasound imaging itself is significant as a material practice, producing such objects or texts as baby pictures and videos. A practice such as carrying pictures in one's wallet is recognized socially as appropriate and not unusual behavior for mothers. By carrying "baby pictures" in her wallet, Josie became a card-carrying member of the "good mommy" club—even months before her child was born. Each time she opened her wallet to show and tell her "baby pictures," she performed her new role. Also, the fact that the images were taken as part of the medical care Josie has sought to manage and monitor her pregnancy serves as further demonstration of her standing as a "good mommy."

Other women in my study displayed their pictures in frames and photograph albums. One expectant couple posted their pictures on their Web site. Another father later included them in the introduction to the digital slideshow that he had created from photographs taken before and after his child's birth, including the first "real" picture of the baby and then the family of three. All of these ways of sharing and circulating ultrasound baby pictures were continued as ways of sharing and circulating birth announcements and later baby pictures. Or understood in terms of literacy, the texts of baby pictures became incorporated into other practices of literacy and uses of text in women's and men's everyday lives.

The circulation of ultrasound baby pictures is an important material practice, even when it involves clicking through the virtual pages of a Web site (or more recently, posting and "liking" it on Facebook). The sharing of "pictures" is met with the writing of cards and e-mails expressing congratulations, the buying or making of gifts either for the child or the parents, and even the arranging of visits from family members and friends who are interested in delivering their well wishes in person. These practices all illustrate the ways in which American pregnancy and parenthood significantly involve consumption, which I discuss further in chapters 5 and 6. For American middle-class families, fetal ultrasound imaging is a ritual, symbol, and—Taylor (2000) suggests—consumer good of pregnancy and parenthood. Not surprisingly, dramatizations of ultrasound scans are depicted in television commercials for Honda minivans, and still images from the scans are featured, in place of more traditional baby pictures, in magazine advertisements for Huggies diapers.

As material objects, the ultrasound baby pictures that I saw had been printed on ultrasound printer paper, which resembles thermographic fax paper in look and texture. At the scan, the pictures emerged from the printer in a long strip, like receipts from a cash register. The baby pictures are printed on relatively inexpensive paper that is not intended for preservation. (This is why paper collectibles are called *ephemera.*) Yet, pregnant women and other family members prize them as precious keepsakes. Layne (2003) describes their particular importance and meaning as mementoes of pregnancies that have been lost. The fact of the pictures provides tangible proof of the existence of an anticipated family member who can be imaged and not only imagined.

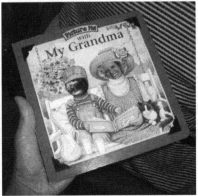

Megan's baby pictures, and especially their incorporation as material objects into other rituals of family and kinship, made concrete her expectations of a particular child and the social relations that will be formed with and around him or her. As a gift for the grandmother-to-be, Megan had pasted a photograph of her mother's face alongside a "picture" from her ultrasound scan inside a storybook titled, *Picture Me with My Grandma.* The book is designed to be personalized, so that the

FIGURE 3.2. Megan gave this keepsake book to her mother as a gift to the grandmother-to-be. Pasted in it were an ultrasound "baby picture" and her mother's photograph.

photographs pasted on the last page can be viewed through cut-outs on each page. Megan's baby and mother appear as the faces of the little boy and grandmother whose story is told in the book. While the gift was a meaningful one in the ways that the publishers of the book no doubt intended, both Megan and her mother also acknowledged that it was humorous in other ways. The grandmother in the book wears long, flowered dresses, ruffled aprons, and her gray hair in curls. She is a stereotype of a traditional, old-fashioned grandmother. In contrast, Megan's mother wore stylish, professional clothing and her blond hair in a current, flattering cut. Also, the black-and-white sonogram that Megan pasted into the book next to the color photograph of her mother's smiling face was a blurry profile of the expected child's head. The effect was, to quote one of Megan's cousins, "freaky."

A scrapbook enthusiast, Megan also collected various items, which she pasted into the baby book that she had started shortly after taking a pregnancy test. These items included fact sheets about prenatal care and fetal development that she had received during her visits with her doctor, cards and notes of congratulations, and narratives that Megan handwrote, describing the members of the expected child's family, including parents and grandparents. When she learned that she was expecting a boy, she began to decorate the pages of the scrapbook with designs cut from blue paper as well as colorful stickers of teddy bears, balls, trains, and trucks—toys that are associated stereotypically with boys. Into the scrapbook, Megan also pasted the ultrasound baby pictures that she had received.

Megan's scrapbook was a document of her pregnancy, recording prenatal visits with the doctor, the ultrasound scan, the family screening of her sonogram video, her baby shower, and finally the birth and first days at home. At the same time, it also was a record of the family life of which she and her expected child are a part. Keeping the scrapbook not only preserved such experience, but it shaped them. In some cases, this entailed a literal shaping of images. Megan not only selected carefully which photographs to place into her scrapbook, but using scrapbook tools designed for the purpose, she also cut or cropped them in various shapes. While some tools cut circles, others cropped photographs in the shapes of hearts and stars. The effect was not only to decorate the pages of the scrapbook, but also to highlight the face or faces of particular family members. Although often taken for granted as mere keepsakes, objects such as Megan's scrapbook and the ultrasound baby pictures pasted into it perform important cultural work in the making of a baby and of kin and family.

Face, Hands, and Feet

The picture itself is an image of the dark rectangular screen on which the ultrasound scan was viewed. The location, time, and date appear in white at the top of the image and screen. Inside the dark rectangle is a gray and white wedge. This is the area that the transducer actually images. The picture taken at my first prenatal visit shows a dark bean-shaped area that is my uterus and, inside it, a smaller, white bean that is the fetus at about ten weeks. Other women in my study had similar pictures taken at early ultrasound scans. Elizabeth showed me pictures from nine weeks, then eleven weeks, of what she called her "bean baby."

The content or composition of fetal ultrasound images is shaped in part by the technology and its uses in detecting and diagnosing problems in a pregnancy. Joan, the sonographer, sometimes described a particular scan as "beautiful." She meant that she had encountered no problems with performing the sonogram, such as when the fetus has lain in a position inconvenient for scanning, and the images were clear. The "beautiful" scan included views of the developing brain, heart, and kidneys, the long bones of the arms and legs, and the spine. However, the pictures that pregnant women took home from their sonograms included images of faces, hands, and feet (and occasionally, also the girl or boy parts). In part, conventions of photography, especially photographs of children, also shape the content and composition of sonograms, making them baby pictures (Han 2008, 2009a).

Layne (2000, 2003) suggests the importance both of footprints and handprints and of replicas and renderings of feet and hands because they symbolize both the general humanness and the particularity of a child. A focus on hands and feet can be seen in artistic portrait photography of children and in other documentary forms. At the hospital where several women in my study delivered their babies, each mother received a keepsake card, decorated with drawings of ducklings, to record the baby's name, birth date, sex, weight, length, and hair color. There is also a space where a nurse places the baby's footprints. Baby books similarly provide space for handprints. Children's shoe stores offer the bronzing of baby booties, or first shoes, as a service to parents who wish to preserve them. Parents also can purchase kits to create their own casts of baby hands and feet, including one called My Little Hand in Yours, which provides materials to create a cast of baby's hand intertwined with a parent's.

When I asked expectant parents what they most anticipated about the birth, they often told me, "seeing the baby's face." In contrast to expectant parents in my study, like Nicole and Joshua, who had given the baby a name, other couples, like Betsy and Kevin, claimed that they could not choose a name until they had seen the baby's face. Pregnant women and other family members often commented that images of a baby's face resembled "aliens." The sonograms did not provide the most distinct or discernible images, but family members and friends still scrutinized the pictures for evidence of Daddy's eyes, Mommy's eyes, and other such inheritances. Many also remarked on the "cuteness" of the baby in the sonogram. Cuteness, however, is constructed through the particular kinds of positions or "poses" that are captured during a scan, then printed and presented to expectant parents as baby pictures.

Two of the pictures that I received at my own twenty-week scan resembled others that I saw during my research. In one, the baby is shown in profile, with eyes, nose, and mouth just discernible. In the other, the baby appears to lie horizontally, with its head tilted toward the viewer for a three-quarters view of its face. Its left arm is held slightly away from the face and chest, and the hand and fingers just discernible—as if the baby were waving. In a similar picture that I saw from another woman's twenty-week scan, the sonographer

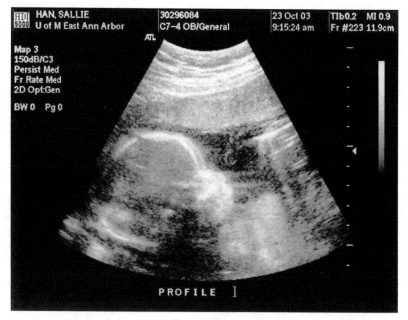

FIGURE 3.3. The image, taken at the author's twenty-week scan, shows the child in profile.

had typed the words, "hi Dad" across the top of the image. During ultrasound scans, images of hands moving across the screen—sometimes interpreted as waves—often drew coos from the expectant parents and the sonographer.

Seeing as Cultural Practice

The importance and meaning that Josie and other pregnant women and family members attached to fetal ultrasound images demonstrate what philosopher Meredith Michaels and anthropologist Lynn Morgan have observed. "Twenty-five years after Roe v. Wade, fetuses have spilled out from the borders of the bitter abortion debate and become a regular, almost unremarkable feature of the public landscape," they write. "They have come to occupy a significant place in the private imaginary of women who are or wish to be pregnant" (Michaels and Morgan 1999: 2). Sonograms have come to represent American pregnancy in public and in private. Fetal ultrasound images appear in magazine advertisements and on TV commercials. They illustrate the week-by-week progress of a pregnancy, from conception to thirty-eight weeks, on Web sites like about.com (http://pregnancy.about.com/od/fetus/a/uswbw.htm), which provide pregnancy information and advice. Sonograms also are kept and treasured as "first" baby pictures and keepsakes of the pregnancy and of the child.

In her essay on the "power of visual culture," Petchesky (1987) described the calculated manipulation of images to portray fetuses as small figures suspended in space, like astronauts. Apparently independent of womb and woman, with fragile, but fully formed hands and feet, they look like little people. The composition of fetal images draws upon still other expectations and experiences, which made the images intelligible and significant for viewers. Seeing is never simply about passively apprehending literal, objective reality, but actively accessing cultural and social realities. It is a process of reading and writing. In the same way that sonographers become trained to look at fetal images so they can understand and know what they represent, we all acquire the sensibilities and skills to see, as members of particular cultures and societies.

The baby lies in the eyes of the beholder. A significant reason why Josie, whose story started this chapter, could see the baby in her pictures—and I could not—is that her expectations, experiences, and especially her relationships with the images have shaped her ability to see them. She reads the images as a pregnant woman and "good mommy" does. This perspective becomes further cultivated at the scan itself as a literacy event. Although the technology now has become both so refined and so familiar that fetal ultrasound images no longer present themselves as a kind of Rorschach test, they do not speak for themselves. When Josie narrated the fetal images, she not only explained what to see, but also educated me in how to read them as important and meaningful as baby pictures. Babies become made through ordinary practices that involve seeing, reading, imaging, and imagining.

Notes

1. As one of the obstetricians there noted, the most common "risk" that they see at the clinic is advanced maternal age (AMA) or pregnancy after age thirty-five, which is associated with a higher incidence of certain kinds of chromosomal abnormalities, in particular Down syndrome.
2. At the specialized clinic, Joan worked with perinatologists, or obstetricians who specialize in maternal-fetal medicine.

Chapter 4

"This Body Is No Longer My Own"

"This body is no longer my own." The first time I heard these words from Heather was when she recalled her initial ambivalence about being pregnant. Heather had felt initially that bad timing had defined her pregnancy. It had not been planned or intended. After taking time off from her studies, she recently had returned to college in order to finish her degree, with plans to travel and to pursue a career as a writer. Then a chance meeting with a former boyfriend brought them back into a relationship. Heather felt happy with her life. At first, because her cycles always had been irregular, it did not seem unusual for her period to be late. After a time, she suspected that she might be pregnant, which she confirmed with a home pregnancy test. Suddenly, she felt plunged "into turbulence," feeling eager and excited to be pregnant, but also anxious, worried, and at times regretful about the changes she now anticipated in her life. On top of the turbulence of her emotions, her first trimester was "misery" in terms of the unrelenting nausea that she experienced. As it quieted, so, too, did her other feelings, she said at twenty-six weeks pregnant. Later, with her due date approaching, we sat in the afternoon stillness after a tour of the nursery that she and her husband had prepared for the baby. She smiled, telling me that the baby was kicking again, then wrapped her arms around her full, round belly. "This body is no longer my own," she said.

As first-time mothers, Heather and the other women in my study found the bodily sensations, moods, and emotions of pregnancy new and unfamiliar. The unsettling of the bodily certainties that they previously took for granted unsettled their understanding of both their bodies and their *selves*. Women in my study described pregnancy as a time when not only did their bodies change, but their *awareness* of their bodies became heightened and their senses became sharpened. Describing to me her experience of morning sickness, Martina said that pregnancy makes a woman realize "you have a body." Betsy, talking over her plans for a natural childbirth at home, said that she had complete faith because "you *are* a body." When, about nine months into my fieldwork, I became pregnant and began to suffer round-the-clock morning sickness, a friend joked that pregnancy had taught her to have more sympathy for dogs, especially their ability to smell even the faintest scents. These days, as the mother of two school-aged children, I not infrequently hear other mothers talk about how not only their bodies, but also their tastes and perceptions changed during their pregnancies, like a like or dislike of steamed broccoli or the motion and speed of a carnival ride. "It never used to bother me," a woman told me as she waited for her daughter at the carousel. "But now ..." She shook her head.

The embodied experience of ordinary pregnancy entirely transforms women's sense of themselves, as I describe and discuss in this chapter. Their feelings *during* pregnancy—both physical and otherwise—were not unconnected to their feelings *about* their pregnancies. Some women found reassuring even the uncomfortable and unpleasant sensations associated with so-called morning sickness because they had been told to expect nausea and fatigue as the natural and normal responses of their bodies. Other women who had experienced no discomfort still looked to pregnancy books for reassurance that the lack of symptoms was also natural and normal. Early in their pregnancies, women in my study frequently told me that their bodies were "out of control"—or out of *their* control—with pregnancy. Later in their pregnancies, with their bodies changing shape and their bellies containing kicks, rolls, and movements inside, women described their growing sense of not one body, but two bodies.

The embodied experience of ordinary pregnancy contributes to the making of babies and of mothers. Yet, the topic has received little serious attention to date. Scholarship that critiques the medicalization and technologization of reproduction seems inadvertently to reproduce the marginalization of pregnant women and pregnant bodies that it criticizes. Where it has been considered, most notably in feminist scholarship, the pregnant body has appeared primarily as a policed body, subject to the prescriptions and proscriptions of medical experts and advice mongers (Oakley 1984; Oaks 2001; Armstrong 2003). Unless they present a medical concern, the physical changes in the bodies of pregnant women tend not to be examined further because they are regarded as natural and normal. In practice, the bodily sensations are treated as signs and symptoms—or trivialized as the side effects of pregnancy or the mere "complaints" of pregnant women.

In contrast, the focus of this chapter is on the "ordinary body" of pregnancy and the quotidian and mundane bodily concerns of pregnant women in the United States today. The embodied experience of ordinary pregnancy is a topic that preoccupies women themselves. In *The Woman in the Body,* Martin observed that "what all women in our society share is the experience of the housekeeping of their own bodies, whose effluvia, demands, and exigencies so seldom appear in schedule with socially organized time" (1992[1987]): 201). Certainly, women themselves experience their bodies as inconvenient at times. The women whom I interviewed sought information and advice—from each other, from books and other reading materials, and from doctors and midwives—on how to manage their physical symptoms and to make sense of the changes in their bodies. Pregnancy is a literacy event for American middle-class women, as I discussed in chapter 1. Pregnant women draw on the images, metaphors, and interpretations offered in various forms of textbooks and written sources, film and video, and electronic media—in order to make sense and meaning of even their most intimate bodily sensations, moods, and emotions. In short, the pregnant body that I consider here is a *literate* body.

It is also a *consuming* body. In this chapter, I consider consumption specifically in terms of the bodily concerns that interviewees most frequently raised—"control" over their bodies, especially in terms of the pregnant belly, weight gain, and food and eating. (In the following chapters, I turn attention to consumption in terms of consumer activities such as shopping and baby showers.) Tracing the modern understanding of maternal bodies from late-eighteenth-century Europe to late-twentieth-century North America, Kukla (2005) observes that pregnant bodies have been conceptualized as bodies that "take in." They consume and they crave. It is understood also that the appetites of pregnant bodies require curbing. Today, the issue of weight is one that receives widespread public attention in the United States as it is defined as both a health and medical concern and a cultural and social concern (Nichter 2000; Brewis 2011). More than one third of all American adults are said to be obese, and a woman's weight during pregnancy has been linked to her child's later risk of obesity (Harmon 2010).

To understand pregnant bodies as not only policed, but also significantly as literate, consuming, and ordinary bodies is to recognize the complexity of embodied experience and of bodily lives. Martina's sense of *having* a body and Betsy's sense of *being* a body both are meaningful in a society that generally defines persons as comprised of a true and authentic self located in the mind, which has a body as its vehicle. The Cartesian dualism imputes distinctions not only between the mind and body, but also the rational and irrational, and the male and the female. Heather's perception that her body is (or is not) her own is indicative of a culture that also assumes the need to manage, regulate, and control bodies in general and women's bodies in particular. Yet, as I describe and discuss in this chapter, pregnant women themselves did not necessarily accept the expectations that have been placed upon their bodies. Even when they did, women themselves recognized it was not just that their bodies did not fit the cultural model, but also that the model itself did not fit their bodies.

In this consideration of the ordinary body of pregnancy, I follow the lead of scholars in the anthropology of the body and the senses, who consider embodiment and perception in historical and cross-cultural perspective. Judith Farquhar and Margaret Lock contend that if the body, to date, has been understood to be "a skin-bounded, rights-bearing, communicating, experience-collecting, biomechanical entity," then a new understanding of *bodies* as "historically contingent, deeply informed by culture, discourse, and the political" is being developed today (2007: 2). In particular, they argue, "this is no longer the body that stands in a tidy contrastive relationship with the mind" (2). They assert that a body cannot be approached as either "a natural self-contained entity organized by mechanically functioning internal organs" or as "the site of will and personality" (2). "To make bodies a topic for anthropological, humanistic, sociological, and historical research is to ask how human life can be and has been constructed, imagined, subjectively known—in short, lived" (2). Farquhar and Lock particularly credit the work of Michel Foucault for calling attention to "the domain of the taken for granted, the mundane records and routines that fill everyday life, the disciplinary protocols that quietly maintain the (historically contingent) normal" (2007: 8).

Kathryn Geurts observes, "In the West, we often treat the domain of sensation and perception as definitively precultural and eminently natural, one of the most basic of the human psychobiological systems" (2002: 3). In contrast, anthropologists have been engaged in studies that reveal the diversity of beliefs and behaviors concerning the body and the senses. Even the number of senses, which Americans take for granted as given—seeing, hearing, tasting, smelling, and touching—varies cross-culturally. In her ethnography on child socialization in an Anlo-Ewe village in Ghana, Geurts found that local women and men emphasized the significance of a sixth sense—what we might call balance—that underscored their ideas and practices of childbirth and child rearing and the feelings that surround their experiences of pregnancy itself.

Duden (1999) reminds us that the bodily sensations that European and American women take for granted as natural and normal today emerge from particular cultural and historical contexts and conditions. "How do we know how women in the eighteenth century perceived the onset of pregnancy? How can we understand bygone perceptions, if we begin our reflections with the assumption that pregnancy is a bodily state that will always result in analogous somatic experiences? In order to listen carefully to the voices of the past, I have to bracket my own bodily certainties about pregnancy—implantation, fetal development—as products of modernity" (Duden 1999: 16). Notably, modern American middle-class bodies bear the influence of literacy. Not long ago, in a class on the anthropology of reproduction, I asked my students—all women in their late teens and early twenties—whether or not it was possible to "feel" ovulation. I read to them from *Taking Charge of Your Fertility*, a book that women in my study had mentioned, which described "a dull achiness" associated with "the swelling of the numerous follicles in the ovaries as the eggs race for dominance and ultimate ovulation" and "a sharp pain" that might be felt at "the actual moment that the egg bursts through the ovarian wall" (Weschler 1995: 65). Many laughed, but a few said in fact they recognized these sensations. One mused that she thought she might have felt it without realizing what it was. In this chapter, I consider the culturally and historically particular experience of the ordinary body of pregnancy.

In and Out of Control

Control has emerged as a central theme in American scholarship on reproduction. Notions of control and planning have been used to explain the development of fetal ultrasound imaging (Petchesky 1987) and the routine performance of Cesarean section (Davis-Floyd 1992). It is a notion more generally associated with the United

States and particularly with the middle class. It is understood to refer to a form of power and of privilege that some groups and individuals have and others do not, but it is otherwise a concept that is
largely taken for granted. Here, I introduce briefly the importance
and necessity of complicating our understanding of control, especially as it concerns middle-class Americans and the ideas and practices of ordinary pregnancy. Middle-class Americans are described as
the privileged holders of control. Yet, they are described also as the
seekers and strivers of control that is either elusive or asserted over
matters deemed trivial. Popular discourse on "natural" birth seems
to illustrate both stances. On the one hand, it is supposed that birth
just happens and cannot be controlled or planned. On the other
hand, it is reasoned that because what matters most is a healthy
baby, it is not even appropriate for a woman to attempt control or
planning for her birth.

Ellen Lazarus (1997) suggests that control and choice—another
key concept in studies of the United States and reproduction—
do not have the same importance and meaning for *all* American
women. It is not only that control and choice are more constrained
for poor women (i.e., they have less control), but that poor women
and middle-class women, as differently conditioned by class, also
become inhabited with different concerns. The poor women whom
she interviewed were interested less in control in choosing their
care providers and more in the quality and continuity of their care.
In contrast, middle-class women "wanted to believe that they had
control over the process as a part of control over their lives" (Lazarus 1997: 146). In fact, Lazarus's analysis suggests that middle-class
women's concern with control is at least partially a response to the
expectations that they *ought to be* concerned with control. "The consumer and feminist movements have created a consciousness among
pregnant middle-class women that they must control their own
lives, that they must assert themselves and make choices" (1997:
150). In short, control is vexing for American middle-class women
and their responses to it—whether they have it, seek and strive for
it, or have it exercised over them.

Control over reproduction begins with planning for pregnancy,
which underscored for the women in my study the importance and
meaning of timing. Considerations included career plans, the stabil-
ity of one's marriage or relationship, and the commitment of one's
partner to becoming parents. Timing mattered in terms of a woman's
age and also her fertility from cycle to cycle. Women in my study
told me that their cycles of ovulation and menstruation, typically

described as monthly, actually varied from as short as twenty-eight days to as long as forty-two days or longer. Doctors and midwives used the date of a woman's last menstrual period (LMP) to calculate the estimated due date of her pregnancy. Being able to report one's LMP with accuracy proved to be significant because it affected how prenatal diagnostic tests were interpreted, such as the measurements of the fetus taken at the twenty-week ultrasound scan, and when a pregnancy was considered "overdue" and became recommended for a Cesarean delivery.

While women cannot control their cycles, they are expected to manage them—in particular, by "charting," or keeping track of bodily signs of fertility as a method of birth control and family planning. Martina, as a committed Roman Catholic, would not use what she called artificial birth control, like the pill, and instead studied natural family planning as promoted in contemporary church teaching. Brett had become interested in charting, first as an alternative to the pill, which she had been taking, then as planning for a pregnancy. In addition to recording her body temperature at waking every morning, she said the charting also required taking note of cervical fluid and checking the cervix, by touch, to chart its position. Charting, as I suggested in chapter 1, is a literacy practice that gives sense and meaning to women's bodily sensations. For women in my study, planning a pregnancy involved perceiving and then interpreting dull achiness and sharp pain as signs of fertility, and developing a level of intimacy with their own bodies that they might not have imagined previously.

Pregnancy, as women in my study described it, involves a loss of control over one's body, both in terms of behavior and appearance. Cravings and other changes in appetite were among the first symptoms that women experienced in their pregnancies. During her first trimester of pregnancy, Dana experienced dramatic changes in her appetite. "Before I was pregnant, I ate only whole foods—nothing processed, nothing out of a can," she told me. "When I became pregnant, I couldn't eat my staple things, like asparagus. If I even thought about it, it made me want to throw up. I was eating Kraft dinner and Jell-O and white bread—all these things that I normally would never touch, but they were the only things that seemed like they would stay down." As an obstetrician, Dana advised pregnant women on nutrition. Now, as a pregnant woman herself, she found that her appetite had taken on "a life of its own." "It was really odd just to feel completely out of control of my eating patterns and my eating choices," she said.

Brett, a graduate student, initially lost weight due to the nausea that she had experienced early in the pregnancy, but at nineteen weeks pregnant, she described an overall feeling of "heaviness." Physically, she had regained her weight and then some. Brett articulated connections between changes that she felt physically and emotionally. She described "feeling uncoordinated" in general. "I'm dropping things more in the kitchen," she told me. "I almost fell over because I lost my sense of balance. I equate it with being like teenage boys, or teenagers in general, and their growth spurt. It's a strange sense, especially for someone who's used to playing sports, to feel so out of control." Brett also noted that her breasts were enlarged and felt sensitive and tender to the touch. Her physical heaviness and lack of coordination were linked to a more general feeling of unbalance that caused her to react strongly in terms of her emotions. "You don't know whether it's stress from graduate school or whatever it is. You're kind of lost to the emotion. It just overcomes you," she said. Brett said she had had outbursts and meltdowns with her husband, who in turn had felt frustrated with her moodiness. "I think men always write women off as being more emotional, but it's really an amazing experience," she said. "You both know all these chemicals are going, so you just leave it at that. From reading, I get the sense that pregnant women are on a constant roller coaster."

At sixteen weeks pregnant, Sharon described herself as "acting so weird" during her first trimester. Smells like her dog's food repulsed her. She had no appetite for the foods that she typically enjoyed. A self-described energetic and peppy type, Sharon said she had been sleeping ten to twelve hours a night. "I just feel like I've been run over by a truck." These bodily sensations were reminders that "I've got a passenger on board," she said. "I feel happy, but apprehensive about having a child," Sharon told me. "There is a lot of change that I am not happy about." Although her pregnancy had not begun to show, she found that her pants no longer fit right. She felt self-conscious about "getting bigger in the chest," so she preferred to wear loose-cut shirts and sweaters. "It just feels unnatural," she explained. Before she became pregnant, Sharon still had the slim and petite build of the gymnast that she had been as a child. She had run regularly until the physical signs and symptoms of pregnancy during the first trimester—including nausea, fatigue, and soreness in her breasts—made exercise uncomfortable. In addition, her husband, parents, and other family members had urged her to take it easy. Sharon, who held two master's degrees and previously worked as a city planner, described herself to me as oriented toward control and planning in her life. Now, she confessed, "I hate not having control."

I noted that interviewees not infrequently apologized to me for "complaining" about their nausea, fatigue, and other physical discomforts during pregnancy. Danielle Bessett reads this in terms of "the dominant cultural discourse of 'maternal sacrifice,' which suggests that good mothering is based on sacrifice for, and identification with, fetal interests" (2010: 373). The women whom I interviewed, like the women in Bessett's study, reasoned that they had no cause to complain because their symptoms were temporary. More important, they were signs that the pregnancy was healthy. "The rationale on which this sacrifice rested was the idea of the productive symptom. Just as some symptoms could reveal danger to the fetus, other symptoms reflected the needs of the fetus. Familiar, "normal" pregnancy symptoms comprised part of the generally productive process of pregnancy and could even be understood to make specific contributions to the well-being of the fetus" (2010: 373)

Not all women in my study described the loss of control over their bodies in negative terms. "This is out of my control," Betsy told me. "I need to trust in my body." Of all the women whom I interviewed, Betsy talked most about "the body's own knowledge" and its "innate ability" in pregnancy and birth. She was one of two women in my study who were planning a birth at home. Her traditionally trained midwives, Faith and Radha, whose prenatal visits I observed for one month during fieldwork, did not prescribe fetal ultrasound imaging or other kinds of prenatal diagnostic tests "without cause." Doctors and certified nurse-midwives routinely recommended sonograms and other screenings, and regularly used a Doppler device to hear the fetal heartbeat, which Faith and Radha rarely ever used. Instead, they listened to their clients, like Betsy, describe their physical and emotional feelings, palpated with their hands a woman's belly, measured its circumference with a tape measure, and occasionally used a fetascope (like a stethoscope) to hear the fetal heartbeat. Although Betsy had experienced problems with her weight as a child and a "complicated" relationship with food during her teens, she told me, "I actually enjoy getting bigger now because I know it means everything is fine." She viewed the changing shape of her body as a "natural" sign of the health of her pregnancy and her child.

"In all those books, they say a lot of people have a hard time giving up their figure—I didn't have that problem at all," Martina told me. Like Sharon, Martina shared the sense that this was not her own "natural" body, but unlike Sharon, she seemed to enjoy "trying on" a different shape. "It's so funny that I have this stomach," she remarked, laughing. "I could be a guy with a beer gut." Teased as a child about being "skinny" and a "toothpick," Martina admitted that she liked the way that her fuller and rounder pregnant body looked. Like Betsy, she viewed her changing shape as a sign of health. "I think it's really neat," Martina said. "Like, right now, you're sitting there, you're not really aware that you have a pancreas or a liver. That's how it kind of is with the kid. You're here and then there's this other there that you don't really notice a lot, unless it moves."

The Pregnant Belly

When I asked women in my study about the physical changes in their bodies and being out of control, talk turned inevitably to their shape. This is not surprising given the equation of appearance, morality, and health among American middle-class women in particular. In their talk, the belly became the particular focus for women in my study. Flat stomachs and toned abdominal muscles are prized today as signs of fitness among American middle-class women, who engage in diet and exercise to achieve "abs of steel," as one popular fitness program promised. Brett and Sharon described receiving advice from their doctors specifically not to do crunches or sit-ups or other such exercises that are said to strengthen abdominal muscles and therefore to "flatten" the stomach. They and other women in my study observed that pregnancy is a time when it actually is acceptable to have a belly.

Kerri contrasted what she called her basketball belly at thirty-six weeks pregnant with her belly earlier in the pregnancy, when it had "the too many cookies look." At about four months pregnant, I recall meeting a professor whom I had not seen in several months and blurting the news of my pregnancy to her because I suddenly felt self-conscious about the way that my t-shirt barely covered my stomach. For Kerri and for myself, it seemed important to be recognized as pregnant, not as overweight. A pregnant belly, unlike a fat belly, is regarded as a sign of health and wellness. Doctors and midwives measured the pregnant belly with a tape measure to track the baby's growth. Martina's doctor remarked to me that the "design of nature" was such that the belly's measurement in centimeters corresponded with the number of weeks in the pregnancy—thirty-six centimeters from the pubic bone to the top of the uterus, just under the ribs, at thirty-six weeks.

Changes in the belly were remarked upon when meeting with family members and friends. Brett and Martina mentioned the fascination that they held especially for their younger, unmarried sisters, who touched their pregnant bellies. A pregnant belly is considered special. Women themselves noted when they first began to detect changes in their bellies privately, usually in the form of what some women euphemistically called softness in their middles, and when they began truly to show publicly that they were pregnant, typically around five or six months for the first-time mothers in my study. Not all of the attention given to the pregnant belly is wanted. Being visibly pregnant with a belly "seems to make you public property," as a woman commented in a birthing class that I attended. Women in my study all had received congratulations, compliments on how well they looked, and queries about whether they were expecting a boy or a girl. They had heard stories, too, about strangers touching pregnant women's bellies without permission. For the most part, women whom I interviewed all found others to be respectful. Audra, however, found particularly upsetting the camaraderie that casual acquaintances assumed with her. A public health educator, she complained to me about the unwanted attention that she and her belly received in the workplace, from colleagues whom she felt should act professionally about her pregnancy.

Davis-Floyd (1994), in a study of educated, professional American middle-class women, found that the pregnant body posed a problem to the conception of self that the women in her study took for granted. First, the visibility of the pregnant body "entails a violation of the conceptual boundary separating these personal and professional realms of life," she noted. "Sexuality and children are plainly part of the personal domain; they do not belong at work" (1994: 206). Second, the out-of-control experiences of pregnancy (and, later, birth) seem to bring to the fore the biological and personal aspects of the self, which women cultivate as cultural and professional. Although women in my study shared the news of their pregnancy with their family members and friends even in the first few weeks, in general, they preferred to "be discreet," as Rebecca said, especially in the workplace.

Yet, in recent years, there also has been the growing visibility of pregnancy—that is, of pregnant bodies and bellies—in popular culture. Images of pregnant bodies, clothed and unclothed, now appear in commercial and artistic photography. As a symbol of pregnancy, the pregnant belly has become capitalized upon in advertisements not only for goods and services related directly to childbearing and child rearing, such as fertility clinics, but also for other products such as life insurance and automobiles. Feminist scholars suggest that pregnancy itself has come to be considered a good or service that can be traded—a process that they call the commodification of pregnancy—in the context of reproductive technologies such as assisted conception. Media reports tend to speculate upon and sensationalize the new choices being made available to parents. Notably, the application of preimplantation genetic diagnosis, which had been developed to screen the embryos of parents with known genetic diseases, has led to talk about designer babies. Sandra Matthews and Laura Wexler (2000) suggest that there has been growing popular awareness of pregnancy as a commodity, and of the pregnant belly as precious, like the diamond ring and earrings that actress Demi Moore, otherwise nude, wore on the cover of *Vanity Fair.* The pregnant belly itself is "vividly unadorned" and the actress holds it in her arms "exactly as she might a bulging shopping bag from some boutique" (Matthews and Wexler 2000: 203). By extension, they suggest that the baby she gets has become "a perfectible product" and "the ultimate capitalist trophy" (203).

The perfectibility of both children and of women's bodies has extended to the pregnant belly itself. There are now a number of commercially manufactured and marketed products to be used on the belly to enhance its appearance. Lotions and creams are advertised as preventing or even erasing so-called stretch marks, or the scars caused by the skin's stretching. Balms and massage oils are said to relieve and soothe another condition that some pregnant women have called belly itch, which was a mild discomfort that some women described as a result of the skin's stretching. While working part-time in a store that sold pregnancy clothing, I observed the trend toward form-fitting fashions that show the "bump" to maximum advantage. Although they were not necessarily styles of clothing that appealed to all of the women shopping at the store, ribbed sweaters and fitted jersey knit tops were advertised as staples for a pregnant woman's wardrobe.

Some of the women in my study had their partners photograph them at regular intervals during the pregnancy to document the growing belly. Dana and Betsy both posed for pregnant pictures with a professional photographer, a former midwife and doula who described her specialty as pregnancy, birth, and newborn photography. (In addition, Betsy had her home birth photographed.) With the aid of a few close friends, Betsy also created a plaster cast of her belly a few weeks before she delivered her daughter. During my fieldwork,

I met other women who also created belly casts as "souvenirs" of their pregnancies and especially of their pregnant bellies. Another way to understand these activities is as the production of texts akin to the fertility charts and notes that I described and discussed in chapter 1. Or, like the ultrasound baby pictures that I considered in chapter 3, these texts become incorporated into other practices of literacy and uses of text through which women make sense and meaning of their embodied experience of ordinary pregnancy.

Weighing In

The women in my study were all not necessarily concerned with perfection, but in general they believed in perfectibility. In interviews, they talked to me about not only what was good, but also what was better—that is, better for their own health and well-being, and better for the child that they expected. To this end, they sought information and advice from other women, doctors and midwives, and written sources such as pregnancy books. When I asked women in my study about what they were doing and how they were feeling, talk turned inevitably to weight gain and other issues of food and eating.

Americans in general receive mixed messages about what is healthy weight. Even while they are advised about an epidemic of obesity, they are cautioned also about the dangers of dieting and of eating disorders among women and men. Weight is regarded as an index of health and wellness in general. Overweight places adults and children at higher risk for developing diabetes and heart disease. At the same time, I have heard parents, returning from a well child visit, proudly describe their child's height and weight as "ninety-fifth percentile" or even "off the charts."

Pregnant women in my study received the message that they needed to gain enough, but not too much weight. However, it was not always clear what was enough or too much. (Indeed, as I discuss below, the guidelines on weight gain during pregnancy were revised recently with an aim toward more clarity.) For some women, too much weight gain meant complications, like gestational diabetes, "big" babies, and difficult births.[1] For other women, it implied the challenges of "losing all the baby weight" after the birth. On the one hand, there is a popular notion that pregnancy entails "eating for two." On the other hand, anthropologist Mimi Nichter (2000) notes that "having kids" is blamed for long-term weight gain. In a study of teenaged girls and dieting, Nichter found that the girls attributed the physical shape of their mothers, when overweight, in part to pregnancy. When fifteen-year-old Connie described her mother as "short and fat," she quickly added, "That's probably my fault and my mother's because after she got pregnant she didn't lose weight very easily" (Nichter 2000: 107). Nichter noted that girls in her study had looked at photographs of their mothers as teenagers and listened to their mothers talk about what they had been like before becoming mothers. "Observations of this type led some girls to say that they didn't want to have children because they were afraid they'd end up fat like their mothers and other women they knew" (2000: 107).

Several women in my study expressed both their distaste and their disapproval of overweight. Typically, this was described in terms of women's own feelings about their own bodies, such as Sharon's anticipation of resuming her exercise regimen after the birth. Indeed, Dana said that as an obstetrician herself, what she found particularly frustrating "is how much women blame obesity on pregnancy. They identify it as that moment—when they went through their pregnancy—as the time when their weight went up, and it changed forever. I don't believe that. It's diet and exercise choices through pregnancy." She admitted, "I have a horrible prejudice against obesity. It's not just that I don't like it—I'm really judgmental." Living and working in Michigan, where rates of obesity are high, she explained, "It causes so many health problems, and it makes every health problem more difficult to treat."

Nevertheless, Dana expressed sympathy over what she called the "cultural stuff," which she said caused women to eat out of control. "There's so much emphasis on body image and being thin that even women who don't have a weight problem don't [maintain exercise and eating habits during pregnancy] because they already restrict themselves in so many ways," she said. "I think it has a lot to do with women feeling under pressure constantly when they're not pregnant to avoid certain kinds of food and suddenly feeling like pregnancy is their license to eat badly." From Dana's perspective, American women eat "out of control" during pregnancy because they face enormous pressure to eat "in control" during the rest of their (nonpregnant) lives.

If American middle-class women seem to have an "obsession" with their weight, as some women in my study had remarked to me, then doctors and midwives seem equally obsessed. During pregnancy, doctors and midwives pay particular attention to excessive weight gain as a sign of gestational diabetes or preeclampsia.[2] When

I talked with women about weight gain in pregnancy, many described weight as a *cause* of the two conditions, which are unrelated sicknesses. A few, like Nicole, with her master's degree in biology, recognized that this is not necessarily the case, but the information and advice that doctors and midwives provided during prenatal visits did nothing to correct this impression. Women's weight gain was recorded regularly at prenatal visits with doctors and midwives, who sometimes commented on a gain that seemed too much or too little. This typically led to a conversation about nutrition, exercise, and overall well-being or lifestyle during pregnancy. Some women laughed and jokingly commented on the weigh-in and not wanting to know how much they had gained, or explained in advance such reasons as the holidays, family gatherings, or cravings for milkshakes.

At prenatal visits with Faith and Radha, the independent midwives, pregnant women checked their own weight on the scale in the bathroom. They also checked their own urine samples, dipping a test strip into the cup and comparing it against a chart that interpreted the results. The urine tests were used to monitor the levels of blood sugar, a possible sign of gestational diabetes, and of protein, an indicator for preeclampsia. The nurse-midwives at both the university medical center and the community hospital also asked women to check their own urine samples. I observed, however, that the nurses who led patients to the exam rooms were responsible for the weigh-in. They recorded these numbers in addition to heart rate and pulse on a medical chart. Faith and Radha emphasized to me that even in such seemingly trivial practices were lurking larger issues about control and, especially, trust in women. That is, women were trusted not only to test themselves correctly, but also to record their results—including their weight gain—honestly.

Medical research today demonstrates the effects of weight on the health and well-being of pregnant women and children. The severity of conditions like gestational diabetes and preeclampsia demands serious concern. However, it ought to be noted that researchers themselves have raised questions about whether prenatal medical care—including the information and advice given to pregnant women from a range of sources, including pregnancy books and other written materials—in fact adequately addresses these problems. In his critique of prenatal medical care in the United States, Strong, an obstetrician, contends: "The entire system of prenatal care that American mothers have inherited has been shaped in large measure by our historical obsession with preeclampsia. The general frequency of prenatal care visits and the activities that persist to this day during a routine prenatal examination are geared toward the detection of this disease. But there's one problem with this strategy: prenatal care does nothing to reduce the occurrence of preeclampsia. In fact, its incidence is no different now than it's ever been" (2000: 16).

What, then, is the purpose of prenatal medical care? Or what purpose does it serve? An important critique that it deflects attention—and resources—from the *social* determinants of maternal and infant health. Medical historian Thomas McKeown, writing more than thirty years ago, observed: "The public believes that health depends primarily on intervention by the doctor and that the essential requirement for health is the early discovery of disease" (2010[1978]: 67). McKeown emphasized the role that public investments in safer food and water played historically in raising life expectancy and lowering infant mortality, which he claimed were equally if not more significant than medical and technological interventions. Today, individuals are held responsible for the healthy (or unhealthy) lifestyle choices that they make. Pregnant women become especially vulnerable to policing—not only on the grounds of protecting their bodies, but also the fetal bodies that they also are said to contain (Oakley 1984; Michaels and Morgan 1999; Oaks 2001; Armstrong 2003; Dubow 2011).

The framing of weight as a problem in pregnancy clearly emerges as much from historical and cultural concerns as from medical and scientific observation and study. In fact, advice concerning a pregnant woman's weight gain has been varied. I learned from a Japanese midwife that Japanese women are advised to gain no more than fifteen to twenty pounds. "Compared to twenty years ago, pregnant women today are taller in height, have less weight gain, and have smaller waists," the Japanese daily newspaper, *Asahi Shinbun*, commented in an article published on June 1, 2003. "They have become slim and beautiful."

In the United States, advice on weight gain has changed over time. The 1967 edition of *Prenatal Care* recommends—for all women— a maximum weight gain of twenty pounds, which is considered the lower end of the range today. At the time of my fieldwork, in 2003, American women were being advised that their prepregnancy weight determines the amount of weight that they should gain during pregnancy. Heavier women are advised to gain less weight (about twenty pounds or less) while women considered underweight were advised to gain more (about thirty pounds or more). Several women in my study had received from their doctors or midwives a guide to prenatal care services at the hospital. Titled *You, Your Baby, & Us*, it emphasized to pregnant women that "it is normal to gain between 25 and 37 additional pounds during pregnancy." Information was included that outlined the reasons for weight gain. Interestingly, the weight gain was mapped onto locations in her body, such as two pounds in the breasts, six to eight pounds of additional blood and fluids, and two pounds of amniotic fluid. It was noted that "additional fat storage" accounted for four to fourteen pounds of weight gain. Doctors, midwives, and pregnant women themselves considered this the least necessary and desirable kind of weight gain.

Undoubtedly, the description of weight gain is offered in *You, Your Baby & Us* in order to reassure women that gaining weight during pregnancy is necessary and normal. In part, it also reassures women that appropriate weight gain belongs as much to the baby as to them. Indeed, the most important weight gain—seven-and-a-half pounds—is attributed to the baby itself. It is not only the pregnant woman's weight that attracts medical attention, but also the baby's weight before and especially at birth. A baby's weight at birth is used now as a measure of the child's health and wellness, with low birth weight associated with complications in infancy in addition to development problems and learning disabilities in childhood. Citing the work of sociologist Ann Oakley, Oaks remarks that the attention to birth weight "is connected to judgments about a mother's role in ensuring the baby's normalcy" (2001: 9).

In 2009, the Institute of Medicine revised its guidelines on weight gain during pregnancy. IOM noted that in the twenty years since its last major revision, the population of pregnant women had become more diverse, older, and heavier in general, necessitating a reexamination of the guidelines (Rasmussen and Yaktine 2009). These new (or current) recommendations use the classification system that the World Health Organization (WHO) had developed. The categories—underweight, normal weight, overweight, and obese—are based on body mass index (BMI), which is calculated from an individual's weight and height and used as a measure of body fat.[3] (Previously, the guidelines had been based on the Metropolitan Life Insurance tables.) The most significant change was that women classified as obese (with a BMI over 30.0) ought to gain no more than 11 to 20 pounds during their pregnancies. The recommendation for women classified as overweight (with a BMI between 25.0 and 29.9) is a weight gain of 15 to 25 pounds. About 55 percent of females ages 12 to 44 in the United States are overweight or obese, according to the guidelines, and IOM estimates that about 70 percent of pregnant women "fail to comply" with the weight gain recommendations (Pope 2009). A subsequent study by the Kaiser Permanente Center for Health Research recommended even more restricted weight gain for obese women that is "limited to 3 percent of their baseline weight, about 5 pounds for a woman who weighs 170 pounds" (Rabin 2009).

The failure to comply as pregnant women implies a failure to comply as mothers. "Health experts instruct women about how to correctly interpret their bodily experiences and how to treat their bodies in ways that will ensure that they have healthy babies," Oaks observes. "Learning to follow this advice is represented in pregnancy literature as necessary for the good of the baby-to-be and for the training of the good mother-to-be" (2001: 30). The abilities both to comply with prescription and to exercise control and management over one's person are traits valued not only during pregnancy, but also in parenting. Appropriate weight gain during pregnancy requires women to see their bodies as not entirely their own. As IOM researcher Kathleen Rasmussen commented in the *New York Times*, "Pregnancy is what we call a teachable moment, a time when women are willing to make positive behavior changes because it's important for their own health and their babies' health" (Rabin 2009). Pregnant women's bodily control and management affect not only their own selves, but also an expected child. Pregnant women are expected to take a child's perspective and then act upon it materially.

Food and Eating

How much weight a woman gains is only one measure taken during pregnancy. What kinds of foods she eats is another. Brett and Martina enrolled in childbirth education classes in the Bradley method, which prescribed a high-protein diet during pregnancy. To evaluate their eating habits, they kept logs that detailed their meals and snacks for at least one weekend. The calorie counting usually associated with weight loss diets became a concern for some women in my study during pregnancy. After Brett began logging her meals, she found, at twenty-three weeks pregnant, that her eating habits did not "measure up" as she had expected. "The first day, my protein count was really low. It was only thirty-seven grams," she told me. "I was really nervous because they say that you should really try to target eighty to a hundred grams a day." Brett had considered herself well-informed on nutrition—in fact, she actively sought information and advice on eating a balanced vegan diet, which she had maintained for several years—but quantifying her intake made her feel anxious. Feeling that her eating habits might not be adequate, she made additional efforts to eat better—that is, to consume the prescribed numbers in calories and grams of the approved kinds of foods. Already a careful reader of food labels, Brett described herself as even more vigilant.

Martina had been eating what she considered a balanced diet, based on the information and advice that she received from her doctor and her Bradley instructor. She was gaining weight at a rate that the doctor approved toward the thirty to thirty-five pound range that had been recommended to her as a woman considered slightly underweight. Then she took a standard screening for gestational diabetes, which showed high levels of blood sugar. Told that she was at risk for gestational diabetes and cautioned about the complications that it could cause her and her child, Martina was thrown into a state of confusion and anxiety. She was required to have a special appointment with a dietician, who advised her to alter her diet, in particular cutting her consumption of starches and sugars, including fruits, which struck her as contrary to healthy eating. For reasons that had to do with being practical in a household of two, and for reasons that had to do with being supportive, Martina's husband, Daniel, also altered his own eating habits to match hers. Still, when I interviewed the couple together, about seven weeks before the expected due date, in addition to their eager anticipation of the baby, Daniel remarked, "I'm also looking forward to Martina not having to do all these special things [and] just be able to go back to normal life and just be able to eat whatever she wants to."

Later, Martina learned that the value of the screening actually is considered questionable among doctors and midwives. In fact, a few other women in my study, like Nicole, refused even to take the screening. At that point, Martina questioned the reliability of the screening, given its high rate of false positive results. The result of the screening and the response of her doctor to it had caused Martina and Daniel enormous anxiety and stress, not to mention the inconvenience of altering completely their eating habits. Martina wondered whether it all had been medically necessary, but added that for her, as a mother, it was more important "not to take chances" with the baby. Martina not only placed what had been identified as her child's interests ahead of her own, but she also both dismissed the discomfort and even distress to herself as unimportant and downplayed the efforts that she had made as no bother or trouble at all. In so doing, she enacts and establishes her role and responsibility as a mother who accommodates and adopts the point of view of the child.

Feminist scholars have commented on the social policing of pregnant women's bodies and selves by other mothers, by doctors and midwives, and by advice mongers who define the dos and don'ts. It seems both that women themselves cannot be trusted and that women cannot trust their own bodies to regulate the necessary and normal weight gain for pregnancy. Yet, pregnant women themselves also come to absorb the values of pregnancy policing. What is especially striking from the perspective of anthropology, however, is that cultural and social expectations become experienced as bodily certainties. When Martina refuses to take chances, it is not on behalf of a concept, but of a baby that is real and present to her. "The entire time, pretty much from the sixth week, I was ravenous. I was notorious in my family for not eating. I never ate, and then all of a sudden, I have to eat, otherwise I'm in pain," Martina remarked about changes in her appetite during pregnancy. "It's kind of different because there's this other being inside me."

Susan Markens, Carol Browner, and Nancy Press observed that "pregnant women's diet modifications during pregnancy are constantly under negotiation as specific practices are weighed against the pregnant woman's wants, desires, needs, and perceptions of overall health" (1997: 361). Brett and Martina both felt obligated to change their eating habits, which presented them both with challenges. In a sense, they were negotiating their own wants and needs against the child's. However, they did not always seem to experience these negotiations as conflict. Pregnant women "are accountable to and influenced by biomedical proscriptions and related discourses of maternal responsibility. At the same time they attend to their own desires for a healthy baby, as well as their own health and perceptions of what will enhance their well-being, which may or may not be in conflict with biomedical notions" (1997: 368). "Right off the bat I'm already being a mother," a woman in their study explained to them. "Granted I'm the baby's mother, but the baby's not here yet, but I still feel responsible and I still feel the care is necessary" (1997: 359).

"Eating for two" or "feeding the fetus" is part of the work of "feeding the family." Sociologist Marjorie DeVault (1991) has considered the importance and meaning of feeding the family, including the provisioning, planning, and preparing of meals. DeVault noted, for example, the significance attached to identifying good buys and especially foods that are healthful. "Virtually all those I talked with emphasized that they chose foods they believed were nutrition-ally beneficial for their families, and most made some reference to widely disseminated nutritional principles emphasizing the importance of a varied, low-fat diet" (1991: 69). Women in my study described their pregnancies as motivation for more balanced, careful, and nutritious eating. They also became label conscious regarding the nutritional content of the foods that they consumed, such as additives. Bridget began shopping at a grocery store located farther from and less convenient to home because there she could buy milk that was advertised as "hormone-free" and "organic." Other women whom I interviewed also mentioned shopping more frequently for organic foods as well as at stores like Whole Foods and the People's Food Co-op, which specialized in food that was raised locally as well as organically. However, buying organic fruits, vegetables, milk, eggs, and meat generally cost more (and sometimes considerably more) than buying "conventional" foods. Whole Foods became dubbed "Whole Paycheck" due to its high prices. This caused a strain for women like Betsy, who said she preferred organic foods, but could not afford to buy them regularly. She and her husband, Kevin, both held part-time jobs while they were attempting to establish themselves. Betsy had been contemplating a return to school in order to finish her college degree, and Kevin had been pursuing leads to break into the music industry. Betsy occasionally expressed to me her feelings of "struggle" because she wanted to eat "better" food for the sake of her pregnancy and her child, but had to "settle" for what she could afford.

The emphasis on the right kinds of foods emerges from ideas and practices regarding food, health, and morality (Brandt and Rozin 1997). The right kinds of foods provide the right kinds of resources for healthy bodies, the reasoning goes, and choosing health is *the* moral—in other words, the appropriate, proper, and correct—decision. Kukla (2005) notes a long-standing concern with pregnant bodies. Maternal bodies have been conceptualized as permeable and penetrable on the one hand, and consuming and craving on the other hand. As a result, the womb—conceptualized as a pure space—requires protection, not only against outside forces, but also against women's own appetites. "Across history, we have worried about what pregnant women eat, breathe, drink, and absorb, and (more or less vividly at different moments in history) even what they see, smell, wish, and imagine, insofar as all these ingestions risk polluting the space of the womb" (Kukla 2005: 6).

The priority placed on organic foods in particular during pregnancy reveals ideas and practices concerning the composition of bodies themselves. Anthropologist Janet Carsten (1997) described the case in Malaysia, where beliefs traditionally have been held that rice, once consumed, is transformed into blood, which then forms the bodies of persons. In the United States, knowledge of biology, chemistry, and other such processes presumably disproves (and precludes) such ideas from being held among educated, professional middle-class women and men, who describe food in terms of such components as calories, proteins and sugars, and vitamins. In practice, however, they understand a pregnant woman's eating habits as leaving a lasting legacy in the body of the child. "Your fetus is what you eat—and what you don't eat," chided the authors of *What to Eat When You're Expecting*. "As you can probably guess, a baby made up of candy bars and colas is quite different from a baby made up of whole-grain breads and milk" (Eisenberg et. al 1986: 18). For the American middle-class women and men in my study, the pure-and-naturalness of whole and organic food seemed to index the pure-and-naturalness of the body of the expected child. Although some women worried about the expense, they still paid the higher prices at Whole Foods in the interest of the whole child. Spending money on the "priceless" child has become itself a form of parenting in the United States, as Zelizer (1985) has noted.

Finally, it is interesting to consider the proscriptions placed particularly on the consumption of sugar, caffeine, and alcohol during pregnancy. At thirty-three weeks pregnant, Martina recalled: "I had a dream last night—two dreams—that I was eating chocolate ice cream. It's kind of scary because I had a dream like this last week. I had a dream I was eating a brownie and I woke up and I was like, 'Did I actually eat a brownie?' Because I didn't know it was really a dream—and I can't eat chocolate." At this point, her husband, Daniel, added, "Well, there's caffeine in it," but Martina replied, "There's not a lot of caffeine, but it has a lot of sugar in it." For health-conscious Americans, sugar and caffeine represent vice substances along with alcohol, which in effect is prohibited for pregnant women in the United States.

The consumption of caffeine in particular has provoked popular concern about miscarriage. However, the American College of Obstetricians and Gynecologists (ACOG) in 2010 issued a report advising doctors and pregnant women that the moderate intake of less than 200 mg per day appeared to have no effect. An eight-ounce cup of coffee contains about 137 mg. Teas, colas, and candies contain much less. Tellingly, one woman described foregoing her morning coffee as making a *sacrifice* for her pregnancy, invoking a term and concept strongly associated with the ideal of mother love.

The hesitation and reluctance of at least some American middle-class women to indulge in these vice substances might reflect concerns regarding the pure-and-naturalness of food and bodies that I discussed above. In addition, Martin (1992[1987]) locates ideas and practices of control and planning regarding reproduction in the machines and factories of American and European industrial production. She notes that the Industrial Revolution represents a revolution in management of bodies in time and space. Sidney Mintz (1986) has demonstrated the particular importance of sugar in fueling the Industrial Revolution, as well as considered the similar significance of caffeine in keeping workers working (Mintz 1997). Thus, foregoing sugar and caffeine during pregnancy signals a shift in priorities from production to reproduction.

Armstrong, in her account of fetal alcohol syndrome (FAS), raises questions about how and why the risk of FAS has become universalized so that "according to the official prohibitions of the US surgeon general, *all* pregnant women who drink are at risk of having a baby with fetal alcohol syndrome" (2003: 218). While not disputing its reality or the severity of birth defects associated with it, she notes that FAS affects fewer than 5 percent of babies born to women who drank heavily during pregnancy and asks, "How can we reconcile this fact with claims that all pregnant women must avoid alcohol?" (2003: 4). Armstrong observes also that the statistics on fetal alcohol syndrome vary widely and that the numbers associated with different populations are variable, with the lowest rates among whites (0.9 cases per 10,000 births) and the highest rates among Native Americans (29.9 cases per 10,000 births). "Because the syndrome is notoriously difficult to diagnose and because there is no biological marker that can confirm the diagnosis, FAS is subject to ascertainment bias—that is, doctors may be predisposed to see it more in some groups than in others" (2003: 5). She argues that FAS deflects attention from the social, political, and economic conditions that ought to be recognized as "risks" to the responsibility (or irresponsibility) of individuals who make good (or bad) choices.

Getting the Body Back

Pregnancy and birth do not leave women's bodies unchanged. Although some women experience nausea during the first trimester that causes them to lose weight initially—and a few women experience such severe nausea that they are prescribed medication in order to enable them to eat—women gain weight during pregnancy,

and some women gain considerable weight that proves difficult to
shed. As they anticipated their births, Sharon and other women in
my study identified "getting the body back" as a postpartum priority.
However, even after their births, women in my study encountered
difficulties. Kerri and Amanda both subsequently had Cesarean de-
liveries, which meant that recovery from birth also entailed length-
ier recovery from surgery. Kerri, Amanda, and Betsy (who gave
birth at home, as she had planned) all were due during the winter
months, which in Michigan also limited the opportunities for new
mothers to walk outdoors—which is recommended as a low-impact
exercise for postpartum women as well as an enjoyable experience
as new mothers can bring their babies with them in strollers, front
carriers, or slings. In addition, all of the women whom I interviewed
at least attempted breastfeeding on demand, which also complicated
getting the body back as the babies asserted their own needs on their
mothers' bodies (Upton and Han 2003). Even among women who
immediately lost their pregnancy weight and slimmed to their pre-
pregnancy sizes, there was talk about changes in the shape of their
bodies, with weight apparently redistributed to waist, hips, thighs,
or other parts where it previously had not been noticed, as I learned
both from the new mothers in my study as well as other family
members, friends, and acquaintances. The making of a mother is an
experience of the body.

Notes

1. According to the American Diabetes Association (http://www.diabetes
   .org/diabetes-basics/gestational/what-is-gestational-diabetes), gestational
   diabetes affects about 18 percent of pregnancies. Its cause is unknown,
   but it is believed to be linked to hormones from the placenta blocking the
   action of insulin in a pregnant woman. Untreated, gestational diabetes
   can lead to macrosomia or a "fat" baby with risks of injury during birth
   and problems with breathing.
2. Preeclampsia, also known as toxemia, is marked by high blood pressure
   and high levels of protein in the urine, which is a reason why urinalysis
   is performed routinely at prenatal visits. According to the Preeclampsia
   Foundation (http://www.preeclampsia.org), preeclampsia is "most often
   characterized by a rapid rise in blood pressure that can lead to seizure,
   stroke, multiple organ failure and death of the mother and/or baby."
   In addition, sudden weight gain is another symptom. The cause of preeclampsia is not known.
3. A BMI calculator can be accessed on the Web site for the National Heart,
   Lung, and Blood Institute at http://www.nhlbisupport.com/bmi/.

Chapter 5

MAKING ROOMS FOR BABIES
HOUSES, NURSERIES, AND BABY THINGS

Lives are mingled together, and this is how, among
persons and things so intermingled, each emerges
from their own sphere and mixes together.
—Mauss, *The Gift*

Like other couples eager to make their new house a home, Audra
and her husband, George, chose paint colors, arranged their furniture, and displayed pictures from their wedding on shelves. Audra
moved her desk and computer into the extra bedroom, to use as her
home office, but otherwise left it unchanged. A crayon-shaped light
fixture brightened the room, which had belonged to a child. Audra
told me she had kept it with the hope of having a child herself. Now,
she showed me the room with a shine in her eye. There were boxes
of files still to be stored elsewhere, but already, this was the baby's
room, with a crib to be assembled, and bags of baby clothes to be
laundered and folded.

Marcel Mauss, in his essay, *The Gift*, considered the relationship
between persons and objects: "Souls are mixed with things; things
with souls." Americans today take for granted a distinction between
a house and a home. A house is a thing. A home is made of (and by)
people. Or rather, it is a thing inhabited by (or with) persons and
their hopes, tastes, histories, and trajectories, which become contained in still other things, like the incomplete set of china or silver
for twelve that a newlywed couple has begun to collect for the holi-
day dinners they plan to host, the living room lamps passed down
from a grandmother, or the crayon-shaped lamp that Audra kept in

the room that she left untouched for the child she hoped to have. Yet, Mauss might suggest that there is no absolute distinction between houses and homes, or things and people.

Spaces, places, and material culture play meaningful parts in the being and becoming of persons (Parkin 1999). In this chapter and in the one that follows, I consider how and why houses, homes, and things matter in the making of babies and mothers and fathers in America.

However, the significance of houses and things cannot be discussed adequately without recognition of how they come into people's lives and experiences. Both houses and the other things that I describe and discuss in this chapter and the next one enter through American women's and men's participation in a market culture and consumer society. Recent scholarship considers the complexities of the relationship between consumption and reproduction in the United States (Layne 1999; Cook 2003; Schor 2004; Taylor et al. 2004; Taylor 2008). Much of it has been critical of the reduction of cultural and social life, especially concerning children and families, to consumer activity. Elizabeth Chin, in her study of children and consumption, argues that "the incursions made by commodity processes into their lives were more complete, compelling, and in some instances more pernicious than ever before" (2001: 4). Discussed popularly as a moral failure—Americans as a society and as individuals have chosen consumption over production, and things over people—Chin reminds us that the orientation to consumption is historically, politically, and economically structured. An especially memorable example is President George W. Bush's exhortation "to go shopping" after September 11, but this is indicative of how Americans have become conceptualized as consumers, not citizens.

This is the context in which shopping has become an important and necessary practice of parenting and especially mothering. Whether it is a house or home, a baby's room or nursery, or the many things that outfit a child's existence, appropriate provision is evidence of a parent's priorities, placing the child's needs and wants ahead of her or his own. It is also a demonstration of a parent's abilities in what I will call consumer literacy or a knowledge of what things are needed and wanted, where to acquire them, and how much to pay for them.

The focus in this chapter is on the significance of things and on consumption as a practice of ordinary pregnancy. In the first part of the chapter, I explore the house and home. In the second part, I examine the things that become acquired to prepare for an imagined and expected child. The theme of the gift is introduced here, with further discussion in chapter 6, which is focused on baby showers.

For American middle-class women and men, the house and home and the things contained within them represent meaningful experiences of ordinary pregnancy. In the remodeling of house and home, families become remade. "The house offers a useful alternative to other ways of talking about the social relations usually subsumed under the term kinship," archaeologist Rosemary Joyce notes (2000: 190). Today, kinship and family are recognized as social and not necessarily biological relationships. The house is good to think with, as Claude Levi-Strauss asserted, because it is "the material grounding for relationship is not blood, but common investment in the house estate" (Joyce 2000: 190). Kinship and family are made from the activities and artifacts of house and home.

Mauss, whose quote opens this chapter, suggested that the exchange of things as gifts is especially significant as the establishment and maintenance of obligation between persons. The exchange is said to transform the nature of the things themselves and of the persons participating in it. In the United States, as in a number of other societies, children themselves frequently are described as gifts. Interestingly, parents also are obligated to them. All of the things that pregnant women acquire for their imagined or expected children are gifts, which transform the things themselves from commodities to manifestations of mother love. In addition, the things that furnish and decorate the baby's room or nursery and provision the child's anticipated needs and wants also incorporate babies into families as material and real members.

Babies Bring Houses

The significance of house and home resonated especially with Faith and Radha, independent midwives who attended home births. Although both women had backgrounds in nursing, they were not trained as CNMs, who represent mainstream midwifery in the United States today. Instead, Faith and Radha described themselves as committed to what they called the "tried and true" traditions of training through apprenticeship with experienced midwives and of birthing at home. They worked independently, with no affiliation to the local hospitals. Faith and Radha had learned early in their partnership that a midwifery practice dedicated to home birth could be difficult to run from their own homes. They rented an office in a small building that was the only nonresidential structure on a tree-lined block. As the estimated due date drew closer, Faith and Radha arranged visits at their clients' homes, but they held most of the prenatal visits in their office, in which they had taken care to construct a home-like atmosphere.[1] The cheerful clutter of plants, pillows, and comfortable chairs contrasted with the nondescript decor typical of medical offices and exam rooms. It was important to Faith and Radha that their office felt "like home" as they wished to create a hospitable setting that put pregnant women at ease, to set their home birth midwifery practice apart from hospital-based obstetric practices, to demonstrate the significance of the environment for a woman's experience of childbearing and childbirth, and to express and reveal something about themselves to their clients in order to cultivate trust.

Faith and Radha laughed knowingly when clients, typically around their third trimester, described the bustle of activity around and about their houses commonly called "nesting." Women who admitted that they had never washed their windows now found themselves vacuuming corners that they previously avoided, washing and ironing curtains, organizing closets and garages, scouring sinks, and even regrouting bathtubs. In the weeks before her estimated due date, Betsy, who was planning a home birth with Faith and Radha, told me that she had been "obsessively" cleaning her apartment in addition to rearranging furniture and laundering baby clothes. Nicole, who was planning a birth at home with other midwives, had begun stocking supplies such as gauze and pads for the birth, receiving blankets and diapers for the baby, and a plastic basin for the placenta. These she neatly arranged on plastic shelves that she had assembled in the small bedroom that had been designated as the baby's room. She also told me that she had embarked on a cooking "spree," stocking her freezer with lasagna and other meals that required only reheating. Faith and Radha saw nesting as a kind of "instinct" and a sign of a pregnant woman's physical, spiritual, and social readiness for childbirth.

"Home-birthing women are acutely aware of how place shapes a woman's experience of birth," Klassen observes in her study of home birth in the United States. "Squeezing into a car in the midst of labor to rush to a hospital, a foreign environment peopled with strangers (some of whom are very ill), is not their picture of an ideal way to give birth. Instead, they assert that place has the power to shape a woman's bodily, emotional, and even religious responses to childbirth" (2001: 97). For Faith and Radha and the women who sought their care, it is not the hospital, but the home that represents a safe space for childbirth. To them, hospitals were impersonal places where birth was treated as business. "Sometimes it is an eager baby who 'decides' where it will be born," writes Pam England, a midwife and author of *Birthing from Within*, a childbirth preparation book that Faith and Radha recommended to their clients. "More often these days it is health insurance which most influences where we give birth" (England and Horowitz 1998: 82–83). From the perspective of home birth midwives, the business model of childbirth interferes with the normal and natural process. England describes a "cascade of intervention," which can start with the apparently benign and minor interventions, like the artificial rupture of membranes to facilitate labor, then end with Cesarean delivery.[2] For women who were planning births in the hospital, staying at home in early labor, until the contractions were frequent and strong, was a "strategy" that childbirth educators suggested for avoiding or at least minimizing the need for intervention.

Even in the hospital, the significance of home is recognized. On a tour that I took at a local hospital, the nurses advised pregnant women that they were welcome to bring items from home, like pillows from their own beds, to help them feel comfortable during their stay. Hospitals themselves emphasized the home-like décor of their birth centers, with monitors and other medical devices stowed out of sight in wooden cabinets that resembled armoires. They also boasted dream house luxuries like Jacuzzi tubs. A woman might be birthing in the hospital, but she still could surround herself with things that evoked the home and all it represents.

MacDonald (2007) considers the complicated importance and meaning of "home" for midwives and pregnant women in her account of home birth in Canada. A planned birth at a woman's home, with the attendance of a midwife, has stood in contrast to a birth in the hospital under the supervision of an obstetrician. As envisioned in midwifery care, home is the "natural" environment for childbirth, the place or space where a woman feels most safe and secure and as a result is able to "relax and let go" and "give in" to birth (MacDonald 2007: 131). However, with the incorporation of midwifery into the public health care system, beginning in 1994, there have been changes also in what MacDonald calls the spatial politics of midwifery. "As midwifery continues to work to deinstitutionalize the location of birth and validate the practice of home birth, it does so now in institutional spaces through legitimate participation and authority in the public sphere as a health profession"

(2007: 130). Like the midwives in MacDonald's study, the independent midwives, doulas, and childbirth educators whom I interviewed also worked from offices that they decorated with great care to make "home-like," preferring table and floor lamps to overhead lights, scenting the air with aromatherapy candles, and bringing in houseplants from their own homes. What always struck me during my fieldwork is the paradox of creating a "home-like" place because it reflects the aesthetic (and incorporates the belongings) of particular individuals who also happen to work and not actually live there. Home is at once a place that is specific to each person *and* a notion so powerfully evocative that even a space bearing little resemblance to one's real home can be recognized to be home-like. However, this notion of home is grounded clearly in cultural and social ideas and practices. MacDonald notes that "the 'home' in home birth may call up images and stereotypes of an urban, middle-class, well educated couple living in their own home or apartment" (2007: 144).

French philosopher Gaston Bachelard described the house as "the human being's first world" (1994[1964]: 7). Likening the house to cradle, womb, and the bosom or breast, Bachelard wrote: "It is as though in this material paradise, the human being were bathed in nourishment, as though he were gratified with all the essential benefits" (1994[1964]: 7). Houses both shelter and shape the people who inhabit them. As a result, the home has been the object of romanticization and of reform. Social anthropologist Alison Clarke (2001) notes that in Britain during the first half of the twentieth century, social workers were concerned with the furnishing and decoration of the homes of working-class families. Their failure to exhibit the tastes of middle-class families in their furniture and decor was interpreted as a failing in morals and values.

House and home and the things contained in them directly concern class as an experience of everyday life in the United States. Class has come to be associated less with labor and production and more with lifestyle and consumption. Today, "middle-class" refers to the things that people have or aspire to have, and through their things, what or who they are. During the first half of the twentieth century, pregnancy advice manuals prescribed the kind of space to be prepared for the baby's room or nursery. "Whenever possible a room should be given up to the exclusive use of the baby since it is hard to give him the quiet he should have in a room that must be used also by other members of the family," the 1935 edition of *Infant Care* counseled expectant mothers. "A bright, sunny room should be chosen for the nursery." The book also included a list of things for provisioning. This advice is consistent with both "a dramatic reorganization of child space and child time" (Zelizer 1985: 50) and ideas and practices concerning class at the turn of the twentieth century. Specially designed spaces, like playgrounds and playrooms, were deemed proper places for children. Failing to provide them, working-class and poor families also apparently failed their children.

Idealized as a private space, the home historically has been a public concern, social project, and "moral endeavor" (Clarke 2001: 24). Today, the "home environment" is the target of efforts to prevent physical injury in older adults and to promote learning and literacy in children. Far from being a haven in a heartless world, the house and home always have been a place of market activity. Not only do Americans spend billions on building, remodeling, furnishing, and decorating their houses, which they have regarded as financial investment in their homes, but in fact, economic policy in the United States long has been directed toward home ownership.[3] A house of one's own defines membership in the middle class. Notably, of the sixteen women with whom I regularly recorded interviews, twelve owned their homes, which they associated with success, but more importantly (in times that they regarded as politically, economically, and socially uncertain), with security. James Carrier and Josiah Heyman have emphasized that "housing is much more expensive and consequential than almost anything else that American households consume" (1997: 12). Whether an individual owns his or her home, where he or she lives, what kind of schooling and other education and economic opportunities are available to his or her children— these can be traced significantly to the continuing segregation by race of housing in the United States. Houses signify more than status and identity. They are "goods that have reproductive consequences" (Carrier and Heyman 1997: 9).

"Babies bring houses," Radha explained. I had been observing prenatal consultations with Faith and Radha. It seemed as if almost every client was either hunting for a new house, remodeling the home where they lived already, or at least rearranging their rooms. Moving house and improving the home were described in practical terms. Faith and Radha's clients explained that their current abodes were inadequate or inconvenient for raising the child or children that they were expecting and imagining. Other women and men in my study (who were not planning home births) also explained the need for a new house in terms of the closeness of quarters, number of rooms, and lack of outdoor area for play. Sharon and her husband, Pete, lived in a two-bedroom condominium with a deck, well suited for a couple that liked to entertain friends, but not what they considered appropriate for a family. They spent their weekends house hunting, with an eye toward finding a home with at least three bedrooms and a fenced-in yard. When I met Brett, she and her husband, Michael, were starting preparations to sell their small city townhouse and move "out to the country" where they could afford a bigger house with room for their family to grow. Both Sharon and Brett lived in condominium developments that they considered not especially "child friendly" or "family friendly." They hoped to find homes in a "community" or "neighborhood" that was. For the women and men in my study, a new house or remodeled home stood for the new baby, the new roles and responsibilities that they and their partners will assume, and the reappraisal and reconfiguration of already existing relationships like friends, family, community, and neighborhood (Han 2009d).

"The birth of a baby most often signals a change in the makeup of the home in terms of its social relations and physicality," Clarke observes in her study of women's provisioning for infants and children in North London. "This most frequently manifests itself in the rearrangement or redecoration of the home as an explicit expression of a pending shift in the composition of the household" (2004: 56). Women and men in my study had undertaken a range of house projects. Each time I visited Greta at her house, I noticed that walls had been repainted, floors refinished, or furniture rearranged. Every time I visited Elizabeth and Ethan at their home, they showed me the progress that they had made on constructing an art studio for Elizabeth, planting an organic vegetable garden, or building a front porch. At first, the couple had directed their energies toward house projects not related directly to the baby in part due to Jewish tradition. Although Elizabeth and Ethan described themselves as "only cultural Jews" who did not practice Judaism, they found meaningful the custom of awaiting the birth before preparing a nursery or provisioning for the child.

However, the couple had begun to take note of electric outlets that required safety covers, bookcases that should be anchored into the walls, tables with sharp corners that could be sanded, and other areas that required "baby proofing"—that is, taking measures to protect babies from things (and things from babies). "Suddenly, I see too many sharp corners," Ethan told me. Although baby proofing the house would not become necessary for many months, when the child started to crawl and walk, Elizabeth and Ethan joked that they already were developing a "baby's-eye view" of their house. In fact, it might be more accurate to say that the couple, like others in my study, was adopting a modern parent's perspective. Ochs and Schieffelin (1984) have commented on the range and intensity of accommodation that adults make for children, especially in American middle-class families. These include linguistic accommodations, such as baby talk, and material accommodations such as baby proofing.

In a recent historical account of children's consumer culture, sociologist Daniel Thomas Cook (2003) notes that advertisers, while appealing to women as mothers shopping for their children, also significantly began appealing directly to children themselves. The child's perspective became institutionalized "as legitimate authority within the context of commercial enterprise. Beginning in the 1920s and gaining momentum and strength through the 1930s and beyond, the viewpoint of 'the child' (both girls and boys differently) increasingly becomes the basis for commercial knowledge and action" (Cook 2003: 121). Children and more recently babies and fetuses have been ascribed "consumer personhood" with significant wants and needs to be met with mass-produced goods.

Women and men in my study took on a child's perspective and took a child's wants and needs into consideration as they remade their homes. House projects represented the transformation of the lives that women and men in my study imagined for themselves. For Rebecca and Tim, installing new doors, painting the kitchen, and replacing the cabinets also represented a kind of closure. These were projects that the couple had been planning when they were married. If they were unable to do them now, Rebecca reasoned, then the opportunity might pass. They anticipated different priorities after the birth of their child. They also worried about exposing a new baby to solvents and other chemicals used to paint rooms and refinish furniture. While Bridget and her husband could have made do with their house as it was, they expected that any house project would become only more difficult to undertake with the presence of a child. For this reason, they expected to spend their first days with their new baby "camping out" in Bridget's brother-in-law's house, next door, while an addition was built onto their own home. It would be worth the inconvenience, Bridget told me, for the baby to have her own room.

Houses Bring Babies

Of all the house projects that women and men in my study undertook—whether they hunted for a new house, rearranged rooms in the home where they lived already, or added new space—none seemed more important for them than the creation of a baby's room or nursery. All of the women and men in my study prepared a place for the baby, even if they anticipated not using it immediately. (They planned for the newborn infants to sleep either in bassinets adjacent to their own beds or to co-sleep or share beds.) Typically, a second (or third) bedroom that had been used as a home office and/or guest room became "converted" into the baby's room or nursery, which itself indicates the relatively privileged socioeconomic status of the interviewees. Even women like Betsy and Martina who lived in smaller rental apartments managed to clear and decorate a special space for a crib and changing table or dresser.

Creating a baby's room or nursery involved decorating the space, furnishing it, and arranging the things in it, like clothing, books, and toys. It involved choices and decisions about the color or "theme" for the décor and the items to be purchased. Women and men in my study spent considerable time shopping, reading reviews in magazines and online, and soliciting advice from friends and occasionally strangers whose baby carriers they admired at the mall. The baby's room is a material expression of parental expectation and imagination. It reflects the perceived needs and wants of the child, and the aspirations and hopes of the parents, all inextricably bound together.

A few women and men in my study, like Rebecca and Tim, wondered aloud if it was appropriate to make "a big deal" of the baby's room—that is, being apparently more concerned with things than people. Even they, however, seemed to see themselves not merely decorating a room, but constructing an environment for the development and growth of their child. Although nobody referred to the room as a greenhouse or hothouse, I noted that women and men in my study frequently remarked upon the number or placement of windows and the exposure of the room. "Sunny" or "light" and "cozy" or "warm" were terms that they used to describe the nurseries they were preparing. Other metaphors of nature were used to describe the baby's room or nursery, which some women and men likened to a "nest." Heather described her nursery as a kind of "cocoon." Interestingly, she had decorated a ceiling fan in it with colorful fabric butterflies that she had bought at a dollar store. Elizabeth emphasized the "womb"-like qualities of the baby's room that she and Ethan eventually decided to prepare. (They initially had planned not to decorate the nursery until after the birth, following Jewish custom.) A gauzy, rainbow-dyed square of silk was draped over the baby's bassinet to simulate the dim, rose-hued light that Elizabeth imagined her child might have "seen" or experienced in utero. Other women and men in my study also attended to the nuances of color in creating the environment in the baby's room. Some selected pastel pinks, blues, greens, or yellows that they considered soft and soothing. Others opted for primary colors for their boldness and brightness. Sometimes, I heard discussion of the merits of blue or green, which are the colors of the University of Michigan and Michigan State University.

Bedding, curtains, wall hangings, rugs, and other items contributed to the atmosphere in the baby's room or nursery. These usually were selected to match each other or at least to complement a theme that had been chosen for the room. Some items were made, but most items were bought. This meant that the theme must be selected from patterns available for purchase. Expectant parents chose their themes with care, considering their meanings. Stars evoked night, quiet, peace, and slumber; it also represented an interest in science for one couple I met, themselves not scientists, but intent on cultivating broad interests in their child. Teddy bears and rubber ducks stood for children themselves. Animals were particularly popular. Farm and zoo animals, like human infants, represent nature that can be domesticated or needs protection. The names of farm and zoo animals (and the sounds they make) also are among the first lessons that parents themselves teach children, along with colors, shapes, letters, and numbers.

Jamie and Martin, whom I met at a childbirth education class, explained that they chose Noah's Ark as the theme for their baby's room because it connected both to nature and to the Bible. They hoped that incorporating animals as a motif in their décor might encourage their daughter's interest in nature, especially an understanding that she herself is a "part of life." Jamie and Martin told me also that as believers in and practitioners of Christianity, they had considered what themes drawn from the Bible might be appropriate for decorating the nursery. They wished for their daughter to be "surrounded" literally with Christian ideas and practices. There was a children's Bible on a shelf. In a corner of the baby's room, Jamie had hung a small plaque that had been mounted in her own childhood room. It featured a poem called "Children Learn What They

Live," which ended with the lines: "If children live with security, they learn to have faith in themselves and in those about them. If children live with friendliness, they learn the world is a nice place in which to live." The care with which Jamie and Martin prepared their nursery demonstrates this sentiment, which other women and men in my study shared.

Megan, interested in creating a "unique" motif, called her theme "Around the World." She covered one wall of her son's room with decoupage, including pictures of famous persons in American history. On another wall, she planned to hang a quilt that her grandmother was sewing for the baby. It depicted peoples of different races and religions, such as a black woman and man representing Africa, and two women wearing burqas to indicate they were Muslims. Megan explained to me that the theme of "around the world" reflected the importance that she placed on exposing her son to cultural diversity. Growing up white in a working-class town, she said she had limited awareness of the wider world. Now, as a preschool teacher, she said children needed "exposure" at an early age.

Lauren, whom I also met at a childbirth education class, described her bright and sunny nursery as "eclectic" because rather than selecting a single theme, she had chosen several motifs. On one wall, she had hung a baby quilt decorated with the artwork of John Lennon, whose cartoon-like drawings of giraffes, elephants, and other animals (originally created for his own son) were reproduced on blankets, sheets, and other crib accessories sold at stores as the "John Lennon Real Love Collection." Another woman in my study, Sharon, also had bought John Lennon items, both because she and her husband were fans of his music and because the motifs were an "alternative" to traditional baby's room designs. On a small shelf near the baby's crib, Lauren had placed a colorful ceramic figure of Noah's Ark, which echoed the animals on the John Lennon quilt. In the corner of the room, a set of figures depicting characters from *Winnie-the-Pooh* sat on a desk, which Lauren proudly told me she had retrieved from a Dumpster. On the wall hung a Peter Rabbit poster. Copies of A. A. Milne's and Beatrix Potter's books stood neatly on a small set of shelves.

Winnie-the-Pooh and Peter Rabbit were popular themes for nurseries and the things that furnished and decorated them. Wallpaper, ornaments, crib sheets, and other items depicting characters and scenes from Winnie-the-Pooh and Peter Rabbit stories are widely available. They and other children's book characters, and children's books themselves, figured significantly in the nurseries that women and men in my study were preparing. They represent a range of hopes and aspirations that women and men in my study had for their children.

American middle-class families attach particular significance to books as symbols of the skills and sentiments considered fundamental to success in school and later in life. "As school-oriented parents and their children interact in the preschool years, adults give their children, through modeling and specific instruction, ways of taking from books that seem natural in school and in numerous institutional settings such as banks, post offices, businesses, and government offices" (Heath 2001[1984]: 318). Compared with the children of working-class homes, Heath found that the children of middle-class homes were enculturated in ideas and practices of literacy from infancy. "As early as six months of age, children *give attention to books and information derived from books*. Their rooms contain bookcases and are decorated with murals, bedspreads, mobiles, and stuffed animals that represent characters found in books" (2001[1984]: 320, emphasis in original). In the years since Heath published her study in 1982, parents' interest and investment in children's literacy seems only to have intensified. Women and men in my study read aloud to the belly, which anticipated bedtime stories for children. Gifts that were especially appreciated were board books, which were printed on stiff cardboard durable enough to withstand the abuses of babies and toddlers still learning to turn pages. In addition, women and men in my study received toy books made of plastic or cloth and attached with parts that squeaked or crinkled, and other educational toys that "taught" colors, shapes, letters, and numbers. In her study, Heath noted that "the only restrictions on book reading concern taking good care of books" (2001[1984]: 322). The parents in her study, like the women and men in mine, described their goals for their children in terms of "'learning to love books,' 'learning what books can do for you,' and 'learning to entertain yourself and to work independently'" (2001[1984]: 322).

Love of reading and love of books were not abstract ideas for the women and men in my study. They talked about their own love of reading and love of books in the concrete terms of the books that they themselves had read and loved. In their nurseries, adults included their favorite books, like *Goodnight Moon* and *The Very Hungry Caterpillar*, sometimes even the same copies that they themselves had kept from their own childhoods. Because Rebecca no longer had the books she had read as a child, she browsed at local used bookstores for "vintage" copies that looked and felt like those she

had loved. The nostalgia of children's books is not only felt personally, but also shared popularly. Even at the time of their publication,
Winnie-the-Pooh and Peter Rabbit stories evoked nostalgia. Today,
the Walt Disney Company produces and markets two different lines
of items based on Winnie-the-Pooh. The "classic" Pooh line derives
from Ernest Shepard's original illustrations for A. A. Milne's books.
The other line features the cartoon versions familiar to the viewers
of Disney's programs. The women and men in my study preferred
the "classic" Pooh. They generally expressed distaste for, and disapproval of, themes based on characters from television programs, like
Barney or Teletubbies. Both in their content (the stories they tell)
and in their materiality (the things themselves), children's books
stand for what is timeless and unchanging in addition to the value
of reading.

In contrast, Daniel Miller observed in his study with parents in
north London, television is regarded as a "bad" influence that turns
"the natural infant into a machine desiring quantities of artificial
commodities" (2004[1997]: 46). Expectant parents whom I interviewed expressed conflicted opinions about television. Most were
regular TV watchers and owned more than one set, typically one
in the living room and one in a bedroom. However, they all were
aware that Americans watched "too much" and shared the opinion
that parents especially ought to be mindful about their children's
viewing habits. They were troubled not only by the commercials
themselves that were aired, but also the commercialism of children's
programs. They reminded me that even educational shows like "Ses-
ame Street" have tie-ins to toys and other products.

Dana said that she "loved" TV and watched a number of shows
regularly. Because she lived alone, she owned only one set, but it
was located in a small spare bedroom and not in her living room
or her own bedroom. Elizabeth and Ethan recently had canceled
their subscription for cable service because they rarely watched TV.
Rebecca and Tim, too, seldom watched TV. In fact, they had relocated their set from the living room to the basement, which they
described as part of baby proofing their house. Indeed, I came to
understand expectant parents' concerns about TV as a form of baby
proofing. Baby proofing involves measures taken to protect both babies from things and things from babies. Expectant parents typically
removed fragile and precious objects from low tables to places out of
a child's reach. Removing the TV or restricting access to it is another
measure to protect babies from things. The television is the material
manifestation of consumption in the United States. It is a commod-

ity that also promotes consumer activities. When expectant parents talked about their preference for books for their children and their ambivalence about TV, they also were expressing their conflicted feelings about consumption in general.

Consumption as Reproduction

Preparing the nursery and provisioning for the child are important commercial activities in the United States today. To furnish their nurseries with cribs and changing tables, and to provision their children with other material accommodations, like car seats and strollers, the Juvenile Products Manufacturers Association estimates that Americans in 2004 spent more than $7 billion. Parents themselves do not make all of the purchases. So-called big box stores like Walmart, Target, and Babies"R"Us, in addition to department stores, boasted baby registries for expectant parents to compile wish lists of the gifts that they hoped to receive for their baby showers. Although all of the women and men in my study were familiar with the "tradition" of the baby shower, which I discuss in the next chapter, not all of them felt comfortable with the baby registry. They cited a range of reasons, including their feeling that provisioning is the responsibility of the parent and their discomfort with the commercialization of a significant occasion such as the birth of the child.

"The nursery, a room given over to the nurturing of infants and the housing of their related material culture, has evolved as a key site of desire and fantasy in the context of mothering in contemporary consumer culture. Popular childcare consumer magazines, recommending nursery styles ranging from the Scandinavian 'natural look' to the cheery primary-colored 'modern look,' promote the idea that a major project of pregnancy is the construction of this child-centered space" (Clarke 2004: 60–61). Couples in my study frequently made decisions together in planning the nursery or baby room, such as choosing a color or theme for the decor. Often, they also undertook practical tasks together, like painting or papering the walls. Men typically took charge of assembling cribs and even crafting new furniture. Nicole's husband, Joshua, taught himself woodworking from books that he borrowed from the library, and built a hardwood dresser for the child. However, preparing and provisioning the baby's room—as activities of consumption—were assumed primarily to be the work of women, who long have been regarded as the shoppers of the family.

Shopping represents a number of contradictions. It involves pregnant women and mothers directly in a market culture and consumer
society that also sanctifies the institution of motherhood and the
literal and metaphorical spaces of children and childhood as *apart
from* the world of work and money. Indeed, as I described above
in the discussion of television, women and men in my study were
wary about what they perceived as the intrusion of commerce into
the lives of children and families. On the one hand, shopping, as
it has been associated with women, frequently has been cast as an
example of irrational exuberance and a form of wasteful spending.
On the other hand, Miller (1998) suggests that shopping on behalf
of children transforms it into a form of moral behavior. It becomes
good mothering. However, shopping does not involve and include
all pregnant women and mothers equally. It constructs the ordinariness of *middle-class* ideas and practices of consumption and reproduction. "The proliferation of consumer goods compounds the
problem: advertisers make mothers feel bad if they don't buy the
right baby products, while advice givers say a sure sign of a 'bad'
mother is a woman who buys her child too much" (Ladd-Taylor and
Umansky 1998: 3). Good mothers buy—and buy the right things.
"Bad" mothers buy either too much or too little, which are signs of
not having the right resources, knowledge, and money.

Gift theory, derived from Mauss, has defined the anthropological study of economics and of kinship and more recently influenced
studies of gender and of reproduction, providing a framework for
understanding the significance of shopping and of the relationship
between persons and things in general. It suggests that the exchange
of things between persons transforms the nature of both the things
themselves and the persons. When the things themselves that become acquired through shopping are given freely as gifts—as they
are from pregnant women and mothers to their children—they become cleansed of their association with the market (Miller 1998).
Or as Cook observes: "By virtue of her presence in the store, with
her children among the racks, and by virtue of her presumed practice of scrutinizing the items she buys for her children, a mother's
intervention effectively decommodifies the item, thus the child, and
affirms their social bond outside the parameters and rhetoric of exchange" (2003: 119).

Here, it seems instructive to compare the experiences and expectations of pregnant women with gay men who become fathers, for
whom Ellen Lewin (2009) suggests there exists an equally vexed
relationship between love and money. Lewin describes gay men as

especially self-conscious about their characterization as conspicuous consumers, given the "shopping" involved in arranging an adoption or selecting an egg donor and surrogate. Indeed, money also seems to validate gay men as fathers in the United States today. The prospective fathers in Lewin's study make a number of financial preparations, such as cutting personal spending in order to save money for the expenses of adoption or surrogacy, and buying what they consider a more child-friendly house in a family-oriented suburb. Children are supposed to be the products of love, not money. Yet, money is what enables gay men to become fathers, initially through their participation in the "market" of adoption or of assisted conception and then through their continuing consumption.

As the shoppers for the family, women in my study also espoused the significance of thrift. Miller (1998) observes that the practice of thrift transforms the meaning of shopping from spending to saving. In part, thrift was a practical matter, enabling Lauren, who was not working at the time, to furnish and decorate her baby's room without dipping into the budget that she and her husband had written. She showed me with pride the dresser that she had retrieved from the Dumpster, refinished, then equipped with a soft pad to use as a changing table. In part, thrift was a matter of not wasting money, time, or other resources. Hand-me-downs were especially welcome, with the givers as glad to pass along their baby things as the receivers were to have them. Dana received offers from neighbors for bassinets, bouncy seats, diaper bags, and play yards in addition to bags of baby clothes. The Internet auction site eBay also proved to be especially popular with women and men in my study. What Nicole described as the problems of "waste"—babies quickly outgrowing clothing and car seats, parents acquiring gadgets and devices that they do not need—eBay seemed to solve, matching unneeded things with people who wanted them. She lauded eBay's affordability and convenience.

Thrift also involves a kind of consumer literacy. Pregnant women whom I interviewed took particular pride in the "eBayed" items that they bought at a deep discount, but were untouched and unused, such as baby clothes with sales tags still attached or baby monitors never removed from the plastic-wrapped box. Finds like these represented the material evidence of their ability as consumers to recognize quality goods and good buys. In thrift, women in my study demonstrated their values and morals and especially their priorities as parents: persons, not things; love, not money; and their children's needs and wants, not their own. Even more important, they exercised their ability as parents to make literate decisions that benefited their children in a consumer society. Indeed, women in my study actively sought information on what to buy from consumer advice manuals like the *Baby Bargains* books, which were written specifically for expectant parents.

Handed Down or Made by Hand

For the women and men in my study, baby things suggested the baby to whom the things were expected and imagined to belong. Books and toys stood for the child who will read and play with them, clothing for the body that will fit them. In effect, the things *made* the baby. Or as David Parkin has suggested, "a person lacks a fixed, decontextualized essence but is made through a social interaction and by taking on the meaning of things standing in a special relationship to him or her" (1999: 314).

Things are important because they are associated with particular people. They represent the people who possess them. This seemed to be the basis for the Jewish custom of awaiting the birth before preparing a baby's room and provisioning for the child. Although Jewish religious law does not necessarily forbid gifts before birth, Elizabeth and Ethan told me that the tradition emerged from not taking for granted the birth or the child. Taylor observes: "This sort of ambivalence toward consumption on behalf of the fetus is perhaps understood, however as (also) a tacit recognition of the extent to which consumption of commodities functions to construct identity in contemporary American society" (2008: 125). She found that pregnant women frequently described the importance of the fetal ultrasound scan in terms of learning the baby's sex and then shopping for things appropriate for a girl or a boy.

The material qualities of baby things also stand for the babies themselves, as Layne has observed. "Baby things embody a number of characteristics thought to be important attributes of babies being small in size, soft in both color and texture, precious (in both the sense of being cute, and of great value), capable of dramatic transformation, animal-like in some regards, and possessing a gender but being asexual" (Layne 2003: 106). Baby toys, like a plush panda or "first" ball or block, are soft and rounded. A number of couples in my study also said they preferred toys and clothes made from "natural" materials. Things bought or given and received brand-new, but intended as "keepsakes" included teething rings and cups of sterling silver and coin banks shaped like blocks or bears of crystal. There also is a category of keepsakes intended to encase the direct material traces of a baby as mementoes of its infancy and childhood. Vanessa, whom I met at a childbirth education class, showed me a glass box containing small silver cans and vials, each marked with engraved letters for "My Birth Certificate" or "My First Curl" or "My First Tooth."

Because they represented particular people and relationships, baby things handed down were attached with special importance and meaning. The women and men in my study told me detailed histories of the hand-me-downs that furnished their nurseries. Cribs, toy chests, blankets, and sweaters stood for the family members or friends who passed them along or crafted them, and the other infants and children who had used them. Things that the women and men in my study had kept from their own childhoods or that their parents had saved were valued especially. These included not only items that could be used again, like books, toys, and clothing, but also photographs and other mementoes. I gained personal insight into the meaning of hand-me-downs when at the end of my fieldwork, I gave birth to my daughter. From her first night at home until the age of three months, she slept in a Moses basket that two women in my study (and their two children) had shared, then passed along to me. The sharing of the giver's personal experience and her practical advice accompanied the handing down of things. A friend passed along not only her nursing pillow, but also her recollections about the first days with her son and her reassurances about breastfeeding. Later, I passed along the pillow, and my own stories and suggestions, to another friend. The circulation of things among expectant and new mothers embodies a circle of support that is both material and social.

Baby things made by hand were regarded with particular significance. Often, they were displayed in a place of prominence. At the literal and metaphorical center of Jamie and Martin's baby room was a large mural of Noah's Ark that Jamie's mother had painted. Nearby stood the hardwood toy chest that Jamie's father had built, which Martin explained could be used first as a toy box, then later as a hope chest that their daughter would take into her adulthood. Both the painting and the toy chest were unique items, which could not be bought or sold. They were made especially for the baby by the baby's grandparents, which also demonstrated the ties to the baby's parents. From the start, the painting and the toy chest were intended as keepsakes. In fact, Jamie's mother painted her mural on a canvas, not on the wall, so that the painting could be kept even if and when the family moved. Although newly made by hand, the painting and the toy chest were things being handed down between generations.

Courtney, another woman whom I met at a childbirth education class, kept a pair of little green booties on a high shelf, out of reach of small hands, in her baby's room. Her grandmother had knitted the booties, at her request, for a child whom she only hoped to have in the future. At the time, Courtney was a high school student who anticipated not starting a family until her late twenties. She had reasoned that by the time she became a mother, her grandmother, with whom she shared a close relationship, might not be living. For Courtney, the booties were a symbol of the close relationship that she had shared with her grandmother. They were as much a gift to Courtney herself as a gift to an imagined great-grandchild. Or as Parkin has noted, writing about the much different experience of refugees and the significance of things to people who are forcibly displaced, there is "a more general process of self-inscription in non-commodity, gift-like objects which, through their association with stories, dreams, and the transmission of skills and status, temporarily encapsulated precluded social personhood" (1999: 313). For Courtney, the green booties resonated both of her grandmother and of the child she imagined and expected.

Annette Weiner (1992) called attention to the special importance and meaning of things handed down and made by hand—especially the things that women crafted, then gave and received as gifts. Weiner called these things "inalienable possessions" because in contrast to other things that can be exchanged (like commodities), they are "imbued with the intrinsic and ineffable identities of their owners" (1992: 6). Indeed, the value that Courtney places upon the baby booties in her nursery arises from her grandmother having been the hand that made them. In contrast, I heard that a local secondhand shop refused a hand-knit baby sweater, in part because it could not be priced. Detached from the people who give them value and without a price, things become worthless.

Women and men in my study received as gifts things that had been sewn, like blankets and quilts, and things that had crocheted or knitted, like booties and sweaters, by women, including family members, friends, neighbors, and colleagues at work. Weiner noted that across cultures and societies, women handed down and made by hand things made with cloth and linked ritually and symbolically to biological and social reproduction. From the perspective of anthropology, the giving and receiving of things on the occasion of a marriage or a birth do not merely celebrate or mark the event. Things are essential to the events themselves. As things identified with particular people, their possession literally mediates relationships between the owners past, present, and future. "When a Maori chief brandishes a sacred cloak she is showing she is more than herself, she *is* her ancestors" (Weiner 1992: 6, emphasis in original).

For American middle-class women and men, a new child is an occasion for undertaking a range of house "projects," from hunting for a new house to remodeling the home where they lived already to rearranging and redecorating their rooms. Women and men in my study directed significant efforts toward preparing a special space for an expected child—the baby's room or nursery—and provisioning it (and the child) with things like books, toys, and clothing. These were not just practical matters. The arrangement of house and home and the things in it were metaphors for the different and new places, which individuals were imagined to occupy in their remodeled lives. Like belly talk, fetal ultrasound imaging, and other practices of ordinary pregnancy, which I described in previous chapters, house projects address the ambivalence and ambiguity surrounding pregnancy and birth. The materiality and realness of the house and home and the things in it made material and real the new family, new parents, and new child.

Notes

1. The midwives referred to clients, not patients, to emphasize the women's wellness and the relationship of care and attendance that they sought to cultivate with each pregnant woman.
2. The rate of Cesarean section in the United States currently is close to one in three births.
3. The global financial crisis of 2008 revealed the deep faith that even supposedly rational economic actors maintained in the home. They regarded mortgage-backed securities safe as houses.

Chapter 6

CONSUMPTION AND COMMUNITAS
BABY SHOWERS

F ewer than twenty people, women and men, attended the shower
given for Rebecca and Tim. It was held on a hot, sunny afternoon
in mid-July in the green, leafy back garden of a friend's house. The
guests sat on the grass or on mismatched lawn chairs, eating pasta
salad and catching up on the goings-on of the summer. When they
discovered that one of the guests was a cultural anthropologist, a
few women described classes they had taken or books they had read
in anthropology. They inquired about my study, and half-jokingly
advised that my "data" would be "skewed" because this was "not a
traditional shower." As expected at a traditional shower, cake was
served and gifts were opened, but guests remarked to me that this
shower was "more personal." The cake had been home-baked, not
ordered from a supermarket. As it was being cut and served, one of
the guests began to sing "The Birthday Song," changing the words to
"Happy birthday to be," as the other guests joined in. When Rebecca
and Tim opened their gifts, they took time to read the attached cards
aloud and examine each gift, giving a squeeze to a plush toy, reading the back cover of a board book. They thanked each guest, rising
from their seats to embrace or reaching to press hands.

This was only one of five baby showers that were being given
for Rebecca and Tim during the two months before her due date.
Rebecca's mother was hosting a "traditional" shower, which meant
specifically that only women were invited. The other four gatherings were described as "nontraditional" or "modern" because both
women and men were attending. Rebecca's colleagues were plan-

ning a work shower, and Rebecca and Tim's neighbors a neighborhood shower. Tim's mother also was giving a family shower that was to include his relatives in Ohio, whom they saw infrequently. Grateful for the care and concern that family members, friends, co-workers, and neighbors were demonstrating, Rebecca admitted that she also felt overwhelmed. (Tim's colleagues, too, had talked about a work shower, but he had persuaded them to hold a get-together later, after the baby had arrived.) "I mean, I would just love to think that we could have all these baby showers and just go and get together and eat and talk with everybody and be excited," she explained. "That's the part that's really fun." What seemed to give Rebecca pause was exactly a reason why other women enjoyed their showers. In fact, it was the reason why family members and friends enthusiastically planned and attended the gatherings. "I wouldn't care if we just skipped the presents at all of them," Rebecca told me, "but I don't think you get to do that."

With family members living in different places, and friends, co-workers, and neighbors differentiated as separate social circles, the number of baby showers being given for Rebecca underscores the significance of the shower as a practice of ordinary pregnancy in the United States today. The shower, as I describe and discuss it here, is overladen with importance and meaning as a ritual that marks the social recognition of new mothers and new children. It now also incorporates men as expectant fathers. Significantly, the making of mothers, fathers, and babies involves the giving and receiving of things as gifts, which suggests that there are meaningful reasons why Rebecca cannot just skip the presents, as she claims to want. Because the gifts typically are things bought and sought, the baby shower is a site and source of tensions concerning consumption and ordinary pregnancy, which is a theme that I introduced in the previous chapter and that I develop further here. A particular source of tension that I discuss in this chapter is the practice of "registering" for gifts, typically at so-called big box stores like Target or Babies"R"Us, which lays bare not only the expectations concerning the exchange of gifts but also their status as commodities.

Practices like belly talk and fetal ultrasound imaging were private experiences. In contrast, the baby shower was a public event and the only "social" occasion given to acknowledge a pregnancy and to recognize the changes in a woman's status and identity. "These events carry tremendous emotional importance for the nascent mother," Davis-Floyd observed, quoting a woman in her study who confessed, "I was so worried that no one would think to give me a baby shower that I flat out asked two of my best friends to do it. I knew I would be devastated if no one acknowledged me that way" (1992: 36–37). Held in the last months or weeks before the baby's due date, the baby shower also has come to represent the social recognition of a baby, especially in the absence of other rituals that mark the integration of a new mother and a new child into a community. In other cultures and societies, rituals are observed after a birth or at the end of the postpartum seclusion of a mother and baby. Although families might observe practices related to ethnic or religious identity, there is no other generally recognized ritual for a new mother and new child in the United States.

Scholars have taken surprisingly little notice of the baby shower despite its importance and meaning for pregnant women themselves. The ritual of the baby shower appears to have become common practice in the United States relatively recently, during the second half of the twentieth century, as pregnancy and pregnant women became increasingly visible and present in public. Davis-Floyd reminds us that before World War II, pregnant women "were expected to remain secluded in their homes, as their presentation in public was somehow felt to be improper. When in public their pregnancy was to be disguised. Even the word 'pregnant' was too pregnant to be used" (1992: 25). As tea gowns, housedresses, and sheltering jackets gave way to swimwear, evening dresses, and business suits, new modes of maternity apparel provide evidence of changes in the expectations and experiences of American middle-class women (Bailey 1992). The celebration of baby showers, not only with female family members and friends closely affiliated with the pregnant woman, but also with male co-workers and neighbors casually acquainted with her, is another sign of the changing times. Sociologist Beth Montemurro (2005), who has written accounts of bridal and wedding showers, notes that the occasions now can include only women ("traditional") or both women and men ("non-traditional" or "modern"). Whether the shower was traditional or nontraditional, the women and men in my study both regarded it as an important ritual.

As a ritual, the baby shower is based on the participation of a community, which symbolically and materially reproduces (and reinforces) its particular beliefs and values at the shower. However, there are competing ideas about community, and with them, competing practices of mothering and parenting. Rebecca received not only five baby showers representing the communities that counted her as a member, but also five *kinds* of showers reflecting each community's ideas and practices concerning rituals, gifts, things, persons, and mothers, fathers, and children. In the United States, where class is experienced as consumption, differences in style reveal differences of class within the "middle class." The so-called traditional baby shower given for Megan, featuring cake and presents from one hundred invited guests (all women), contrasted with the nontraditional open house held for Dana, with champagne and "open mic" performances from the women and men in her neighborhood musical society. The things given and received as gifts at traditional and nontraditional or modern showers all communicated ideas and practices concerning motherhood and childhood.

Emile Durkheim claimed: "Society is people and things" (quoted in Cunningham 2000: vii). However, as meaningful as things are to people, the relationship between them is complicated and conflicted. I begin this examination of the baby shower with a consideration of the question that Rebecca and other pregnant women whom I interviewed all raised about the significance of the occasion. Is it about people or things?

People or Things?

Megan's shower was held in the recreation hall of the church that her mother attended on the outskirts of Ann Arbor, where subdivisions and big box stores seemed to spring whole from former farmland. Folding chairs and long tables covered with white plastic tablecloths had been set for almost two hundred people who had been invited, including family members, friends, co-workers, and neighbors. In the end, fewer than one hundred guests—all women, a few with children in tow—attended. Like many American brides now do for their weddings, Megan had chosen a color "theme" for her baby shower, which her mother and cousin were giving. Yellow and pastel blue, her choices of colors, echoed the colors of the University of Michigan, and were considered appropriate for a boy, as Megan had learned the baby's sex at her twenty-week scan. After the guests had filled their paper plates with finger foods kept warm in chafing dishes, Megan's mother and cousin led a few "games," such as a trivia contest and a raffle, for which prizes like painted ceramic flowerpots were given to the winners.

The main event was the opening of gifts, which lasted over half an hour. The gifts had been collected from guests as they arrived then arranged in a display at the table that had been set at the front of

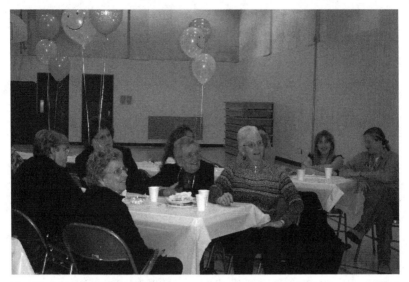

FIGURE 6.1. More than 200 guests were invited to the baby shower hosted for Megan. The main event was the opening of gifts.

the hall for Megan. More than one guest, impressed with the display of gifts, described it as "a store." In addition to the many packages wrapped in pastel-colored paper, there were a few larger items that were unwrapped, such as a feeding chair. Glowing with pleasure, Megan opened each gift as her mother or sister passed them to her, then smiled and thanked the giver. Occasionally, guests called to

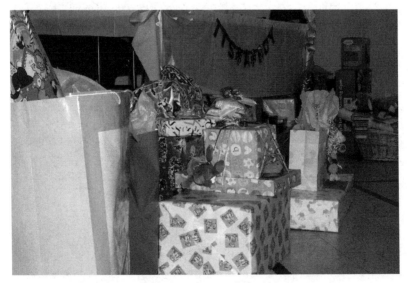

FIGURE 6.2. The gifts on display at Megan's baby shower.

Megan to lift an item over her head so that they could have a better look at it, or stood and took a picture of Megan holding the gift that they had given. Megan's sister kept a list of gifts and the names of the givers. Later, Megan sent handwritten notes to all of her guests, thanking them for the specific items received as gifts.

The giving of gifts today typically involves shopping, and in shopping for a gift, a guest at a baby shower might be guided by her own experience and expertise as a mother, her income, and her own style and taste. Significantly, she might be guided also by a gift registry. Except for the baby clothes, which guests themselves chose, the gifts given to Megan all were items selected from her gift registry. The baby registry itself had included six pages of items that ranged from a bib to a CD player for the baby's crib to an infant car seat that matched the feeding chair and a portable crib for traveling. Megan herself had not created the list, but selected which items and what brands, colors, sizes, and quantities she wished from the glossy "guide" that the store had provided. As a literate consumer, Megan also had in mind particular items and brands that had been suggested to her in magazines that she had read or by other mothers who swore by a particular baby bottle warmer or teething toy. Registering for the shower had been time consuming for Megan and her husband, Patrick, as they dutifully had followed the pages of their baby registry guide. "I had to drag him there," she told me, but his initial reluctance had given way to "talking about the baby" as they browsed the aisles of baby things. Megan enjoyed her experience of the gift registry. It had been an activity in which she and her husband participated together as a couple and an opportunity for them to imagine actively, openly, and playfully the child they were expecting and themselves as parents.

During my fieldwork, I quickly learned that everyone has an opinion about the baby or gift registry. (I have heard similar comments and complaints made about bridal and wedding showers.) Some women, like Megan, not only used it, but also took pleasure in registering for gifts. Other women, like Rebecca, refused it because they said it made the shower about things, not people. Guests at their showers similarly expressed a range of opinions. Some appreciated the registry for its "convenience," as they wished to give gifts that were wanted and needed, without "wasting" time and money. Others disliked it because they said it made the gifts "less personal."

Now used in connection with bridal showers, weddings, and baby showers (but not births themselves), the gift registry originally was invented as a response to the obligatory wedding present. In her history of the wedding industry, Vicki Howard (2006) describes both the

delight and indignation that wedding presents and gift registries inspired in American middle-class women and men of the nineteenth
and twentieth centuries. Like Megan, who opened gifts for over a
half hour at her baby shower, brides reveled in receiving gifts. As
one turn-of-the-century bride confessed: "It is too much fun getting
presents—I adore it and they can't come too many or too often for
me!" (Howard 2006: 116–17). However, a generation earlier, Henry
Ward Beecher condemned the practice of giving wedding presents,
which was still new in 1870. "The minister suggested that presents
were supposed to express a deeply felt sentiment, something possible in a communal, face-to-face world where everyone knew the
marrying couple and their families" (Howard 2006: 117). Now, the
new custom apparently was for everyone and anyone to give gifts,
regardless of their relationships. "For gift givers, registries de-skilled
the gift-giving process, taking control of the choice of present from
the guest, and saving time as well" (Howard 2006: 116). The gift
registry seemed to solve the problems of giving and receiving presents for the twentieth-century wedding.

From the perspective of the gift's recipient, Howard observes,
"registries permitted the bride more control over her wedding presents" (2006: 116). In the late nineteenth century, a customer could
"register" her silver pattern with her jeweler, who then could suggest the purchase of gifts that completed or complemented the pattern, and did not duplicate items already had. In a deliberate effort
to cultivate and corner a new market, department stores improved
upon this service, allowing brides to register for gifts from the range
of departments in their stores, then providing them with preprinted
lists to aid in their selection of items. "The introduction of these
forms marked a shift toward standardized consumption as the re-
tailer now told the bride what she should have in her new home"
(Howard 2006: 117).

The gift registry is surrounded with tension in part because it represents the commodification of ritual goods, which in the past would
have been handed down and made by hand as what Weiner (1992)
called "inalienable possessions." Weiner noted that across cultures
and societies, women bring gifts of cloth, considered a form of female wealth, into their marriages. A custom in Europe and America
was to keep a "hope chest" or "trousseau"—sometimes literally a
chest or box and sometimes not—of clothing and bed and table lin-
ens in anticipation of a girl or woman's marriage. Another custom
was to prepare a "layette" or collection of clothing, blankets, and
swaddling for an infant. Like the things in a hope chest, the items in

a layette previously had been sewn or knit by hand. However, Cook (1995) observes that in the 1920s and 1930s American middle-class women came to see *purchasing* the layette as better quality, more convenient, and healthier for children (as the garments were designed according to "scientific" standards). The selling of the layette, and of children's wear more broadly, in the first half of the twentieth century represents a moment "when the 'sacred' domestic sphere of mothers and children increasingly came into contact with the 'profane' world of the marketplace" (Cook 1995: 506).

Rites of passage, like a birth or marriage, long have involved the giving and receiving of gifts. Gifts do not merely celebrate or mark these events, but are essential to them, as the gifts are affiliated with the people who give and receive them. Although the handiwork of individual items in a trousseau or layette might be quite elaborate, in general, the gifts associated with rites of passage like marriage and birth would have been modest in kind and number—and rich in relational significance. Givers and receivers were involved in ties that were close and direct, if not always affectionate and amiable. If gifts today seem "less personal," as the women and men in my study assert, then it might be because the givers and receivers do not necessarily share immediate connections to each other. The two hundred guests who had been invited to Megan's shower included family members and the friends, co-workers, and neighbors not only of Megan herself, but also of her mother and sister, who were hosting the shower, and the wives and girlfriends of Megan's husband's (male) friends.

Thus, the baby or gift registry exposes the obligatoriness of the gifts that American middle-class women and men give and receive ideally as symbols of love and friendship. In fact, the women attending Megan's baby shower might or might not be her friends, but they are obligated *as guests* to bring presents. Even for the guests who share a close connection with Megan, the registry exposes the strings attached to gifts that are supposed to be given in love and friendship, potentially raising questions about the sincerity of givers and receivers. In "The Gift," Mauss observed that gifts can be given to establish and maintain ties between kith and kin or, as a proxy for war, to defeat rivals. In either case, the receiving of a gift obligates the giving of one—which American middle-class women and men recognize, even as it contradicts their cultural ideal of gifts as freely given and received. In the past, women in my study had given gifts at baby showers, weddings, bridal showers, birthday and anniversary parties, and other important ritual occasions to family

members, friends, co-workers, and neighbors. They could expect to
give such gifts in the future. At present, they were receiving gifts
that reciprocated their own giving, whether or not they themselves
recognized this.

The gift registry also makes explicit the terms of reciprocity, speci-
fying the brands, colors, and quantities of the things given as gifts.
Some women in my study described in positive terms the influence
or "control" that a baby registry gave them over the things that
would be given and received as gifts. Even a few who did not register still shared with family members and friends their preferences
for books or educational toys. One couple that I met in a childbirth
education class had a "no-batteries" policy in order to encourage
"simple" toys with no "artificial" lights or noises. However, control,
as I discussed previously in chapter 4, is itself a troubling concept
for pregnant women in the United States. Rebecca did not register
for gifts despite characterizing herself as a "plan-ful" person. "This
is about the fact that people like to go out and buy baby things. It's
not mine to control and say, 'No, don't get me plastic stuff,' or whatever," she told me. "It's about the fact that people really want to celebrate with you and they enjoy buying baby stuff. So, I should just
let that happen." From Rebecca's perspective, once she asserted control over the things that were wanted or not, they were "all about"
herself as the receiver, and not the giver or their relationship. They
were, therefore, no longer "really" gifts.

However, there is another way to interpret why it is acceptable
and even appropriate to use a registry and to have control over the
giving and receiving of gifts. After all, a neighbor expecting her first
grandchild recently remarked to me, the gifts are *for the baby*. Because a parent will be using the gifts to diaper and clothe, bathe,
feed, soothe, and amuse the child, she or he has an interest in the
things that will be used in the direct care of the child. In addition,
parents have a more general interest in having not necessarily control, but at least the selective mediation of the things that their children can have. Seen in this light, the baby registry, for American
middle-class parents, becomes an extension of literate consumption
as good parenting.

Traditional or Modern?

While bridal or wedding showers were given in the first half of the
twentieth century, both the wedding shower and the baby shower

appear to have become a common practice among American middle-
class women only in the years following World War II. Writers of
etiquette books for brides, however, have claimed a history for the
bridal shower that traces back to sixteenth-century Holland, telling
a story about a woman whose father refused her a dowry because
she wished to marry a poor miller. "Sympathetic to the love between
the two, the would-be bride's friends gathered gifts so that she was
able to wed" (Montemurro 2005: 13). Apocryphal or not, the story
lends the aura of history and tradition to the shower as a display of
love and friendship, and as the provisioning of a marriage (or in the
case of a baby shower, a child) through the giving and receiving of
gifts. Bridal or wedding showers and baby showers certainly carry
the traces of other meaningful customs, like the bridal tea that the
bride herself gave before the wedding, or the baptism of a Christian
child or the bris for a male Jewish child. They also continue the
practice of giving and receiving of things that carry symbolic significance. Howard notes, however, the importance of invoking history
and tradition "to legitimize new rituals and help overcome cultural
resistance" to new ideas and practices (Howard 2006: 3). As rituals become invented and reinvented, they provide the apparently
seamless connections between past and future, reproducing what
we call society and culture.

"Traditional" and "nontraditional" or "modern" were concepts
that women and men in my study used to reference their expectations and experiences concerning baby showers as rituals. Most
frequently, they used the terms specifically to describe whether men
were included. However, they also invoked the traditional and the
modern to talk about gifts and the relationships between people and
things. "Traditional" was associated with the obligation between
people to give and receive things as gifts. It was assumed widely
that the purpose of the baby shower "traditionally" was to give gifts
for the new baby, in advance of the birth—that is, to "shower" the
expectant mother and expected child with the things needed and
wanted. In fact, the shower was important in providing material
support to Megan, a preschool teacher, and her husband, a building
apprentice, who were in their early twenties.

In contrast, Rebecca and Tim, in their mid-thirties, had established careers and savings. "To me, showers are about a young couple who's just getting started out, who doesn't have the money to
buy things, and it's about getting them set up," Rebecca said. "That's
not really us. We're older, we're already set up." Thus, when Rebecca tells me that she wishes she could skip the presents and that

she has not registered for gifts because she does not wish to control what things she might receive, she also can *afford* to do this. A shower like the one given by friends for Rebecca and Tim was "modern" and "not a traditional shower" in part because the guests were told to bring their "presence, not presents." In other words, "traditional" and "modern" also stand for class differences among American middle-class women and men.

While "traditional" demonstrates continuity with the past, deflecting attention from change, "modern" draws attention to change as improvement. Betsy, who was planning a home birth, preferred that her friends organize for her not a baby shower, but a "mother blessing" or "blessingway." The ceremony has become popular as an "alternative" baby shower since the late 1990s. England, in her book *Birthing from Within*—which Betsy had read—describes as her inspiration the quilting parties of American pioneer women in the nineteenth century, and advises women on creating blessing ceremonies that are meaningful to them. The "blessingway" takes its name from Navajo tradition, and incorporates customs from other cultures, such as painting Hindi-inspired henna "tattoos" on the hands, feet, or belly of the pregnant woman or creating Tibetan-style prayer flags that display the good wishes of the guests for the expectant mother. "Even though the rituals surrounding birth have changed with the advent of technology, birth itself has not changed. You, as a mother-to-be, still need to be prepared, nurtured, and 'mothered' by other women," England writes. "Instead of a baby shower, ask your friends to give you a Mother Blessing to celebrate your 'birth' as a mother" (England and Horowitz 1998: 15). Even while acknowledging that the ceremony was invented recently and so could be considered modern, Betsy said that she considered the blessingway truer to tradition because it brought together women in support of the mother, as childbirth has been described historically. In other words, the modern blessingway improves upon traditional ideas and practices of community.

Dana persuaded her friends and neighbors not to give her a baby shower where guests brought things as gifts. Instead, they held what the invitation card described as a "Champagne and dessert open house," with women and men invited as guests. In lieu of gifts, the invitation included a "coupon" for guests to complete as a promise to clear snow from the front walk of Dana's house, do the laundry or the shopping, or provide other help. A single woman with a successful career, Dana had told me that she preferred to purchase, on her own, things for the baby. With no family members living nearby, she recognized her need for time and help from friends and neighbors. At the party, hosted by a neighbor, a large calendar had been set on an easel in the foyer. As guests arrived, they wrote their names on the dates when they would bring a meal or mind the baby so that Dana could take a walk, a nap, or a shower.

By promising their time and help, guests were giving gifts that were wanted, valued, and personal. These gifts were not things, and they were for Dana, not the baby, which allowed Dana to participate in the ritual of the baby shower, and at the same time, to observe the Jewish custom of awaiting the birth before preparing a nursery or provisioning for the child. Many of the women and men attending her party were members of a neighborhood musical society, and the main event of the party was not the opening of gifts, but an "open mic" during which guests performed comic songs and lullabies. Dana's eyes shone with tears as she thanked her guests for simply being her community.

A Public Ritual

Audra compared her baby shower with her wedding in its importance, both as a personal experience for her and as a social occasion in which her family members and friends participated. Invitations had been mailed to almost 150 guests, who were all women and included co-workers and members of the church that Audra and her husband, George, attended. The shower was held in the reception hall in the basement of the church, a stately building on the east side of Detroit. Audra's mother and cousin, seated at a table near the entrance, greeted guests as they arrived, pointing to the coat rack and asking the women to sign the guest book. Audra herself was "circulating" around the hall, accepting congratulations with an embrace and a kiss on the cheek. Guests sat at long tables that were covered with white paper coverings printed with pastel-colored rocking horses. They socialized, sampled foods from the hot buffet that had been set at the far side of the hall, and played word puzzles and other games that Audra's friend led. As at Megan's shower, the main event at Audra's shower was the opening of gifts, then the serving of a large, tiered cake that had been frosted and decorated to resemble a tower of baby blocks.

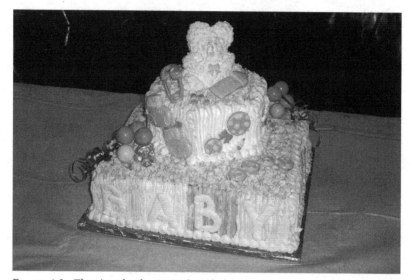

FIGURE 6.3. The tiered cake at Audra's baby shower.

Held in the final months or weeks before the anticipated birth, the baby shower is described frequently as a rite of passage. A number of women whom I interviewed said, for example, that it was part of their preparation for childbirth itself. Having the house cleaned, the nursery prepared, and things for the baby contributes to a sense of "preparedness and capability" that is "an important prerequisite to psychological preparedness for the birth" (Davis-Floyd 1992: 37). However, the baby shower itself does not fit the classic model of a rite of passage as Eileen Fischer and Brenda Gainer have noted: "The three phases of separation, transition, and reintegration cannot be mapped even imperfectly onto the ritual behaviors that occur during a baby shower" (1993: 320). These behaviors typically include the playing of games, the seating of the pregnant woman at a special place or table, the opening of gifts, and the serving of cake, which are activities also incorporated into bridal or wedding showers. Yet, a baby shower more closely resembles a party or reception held after a wedding ceremony than the marriage rite itself.[1] Like the wedding reception, the baby shower itself is not a rite of passage. It is a ritual that publicly acknowledges a pregnancy and socially recognizes a pregnant woman as an expectant mother. As a ritual, the baby shower invites and involves the community, which makes it meaningful for American middle-class women and men.

Although the baby shower can be compared with a wedding reception, Fischer and Gainer suggest that a traditional shower, like

Megan's or Audra's, is similar also to a child's birthday party. "Decorations usually include balloons, and often folding paper items such as umbrellas or perambulators. Childish games which involve simple guessing or luck are played. 'Childish' food and drink are also served; the drinks are usually fruit punch and/or other non-alcoholic beverages, and sweets comprise a large portion of the food provided" (1993: 321). They argue that the traditional baby shower, with its return to childish things, symbolizes a woman's recovery of innocence in a culture where children themselves embody the ideals of motherhood, such as purity and devotion.

When I discussed this analysis with women whom I came to know especially well during my fieldwork or with personal friends, some said that the similarities to a child's birthday party might be appropriate because the shower is not just for the pregnant woman. It is also a celebration for the new baby. However, other women I know have felt that that traditional baby shower "infantilizes" women, reducing them to the status of children. In contrast, at "co-ed" or "mixed" showers where men were present, I observed no pastel-colored decorations or shower games. The showers were more like adult parties, held in the evening, with beer and wine served to the guests. Montemurro (2005), in her study of wedding showers, attributes the changes to the "masculinization" of showers, but the differences seem related also to recognizing the adult status of the expectant mother and father and of the guests.

In other places and at other times, the idea of sharing news of a pregnancy might have been unthinkable. However, in the United States today, it is possible to purchase greeting cards to congratulate parents on the birth of a new baby, to accompany a gift for a baby shower, and even to wish a woman well on the news of her pregnancy. The baby shower is significant as the public acknowledgement of a pregnancy. For American middle-class women and men, conventional wisdom is that news of a pregnancy should not be shared until after the twelfth or thirteenth week of pregnancy, which marks the end of the first trimester, when the risk of miscarriage is highest—or after the results from prenatal diagnostic tests, like amniocentesis, have been received. Until this point, a pregnancy is considered uncertain. The delay in telling is supposed to spare everyone from having to share "bad" news. Some women, however, were in touch with me (a cultural anthropologist studying pregnancy) within days of receiving a positive result on a home pregnancy test. Other women told me that they might have preferred not to tell until after they were "showing," but planning maternity leave necessitated sharing the news with family members and friends, whom the women felt should know first, then with co-workers.

Kerri and Brian told me that an invitation to a co-worker's baby shower was the only announcement that he had received about the woman's pregnancy. This caused Brian considerable embarrassment because it became evident that others in the workplace had known for months and already offered their congratulations to the woman. In fact, it seemed that all of the women and men whom I met during fieldwork could recall awkward moments, some humorous and some less so, involving themselves or other pregnant women. The news of a pregnancy can spread haltingly and unevenly as it is carried by word of mouth among acquaintances that are less close. This can cause problems in the workplace, where it is considered neither polite nor appropriate to take note of changes in a woman's appearance, especially when it concerns her shape. Although it is rude to assume that a woman is "merely" heavy or gaining weight, it is even more inappropriate to assume that she must be pregnant. Contradictory as it seems, it is worse still not to notice at all what to everyone is obvious.

Although the baby shower is typically given for a woman pregnant with her first child, showers are given now for the adoption of a child and "sprinkles" for the subsequent arrivals of other children. Described on the invitation cards as a celebration of the "new arrival," with things for the new baby (or adopted child) given and received as gifts, the shower is especially meaningful for American middle-class women as recognition of their anticipated motherhood. It marks their welcome into the community of mothers. "It makes you feel so special, so loved and appreciated," Davis-Floyd was told by a woman in her study. "And you know these people will love and appreciate this new life you are bringing as well" (1992: 36). At traditional showers, like Megan's and Audra's, the invited guests all were women and typically included other mothers (and grandmothers). Even when the guests were not acquainted with each other, they still traded stories about experiences familiar to them all, like colic and diapers and sleep deprivation. These stories sometimes took on the tone of confessions, in which women admitted that caring for an infant sometimes felt like drudgery. Their admissions rang with hard truth and hard laughter. As writer Anne Lamott lamented in *Operating Instructions: A Journal of My Son's First Year,* her warts-and-all memoir of motherhood: "I just can't get over how much babies cry. I really had no idea what I was getting into. To tell you the truth, I thought it would be more like getting a cat" (1993: 66). In the company of other mothers, women described their loss of independence, in terms of having a child dependent on them, and of having less autonomy and freedom to do what they themselves wanted.

Women in my study frequently described their feelings of "kinship" with other pregnant women whom they encountered shopping at the supermarket or walking on the street. "It gives you an instant bond," one woman told me at a prenatal yoga class. Anthropologists use the term *communitas* to describe the intense solidarity that is shared among individuals undergoing rites of passage, like the "instant bond" among pregnant women. Turner suggested that communitas was a particular experience of liminality, which he famously described as a state of being betwixt and between. At the baby shower, which is given for an individual, not a group, communitas seems significantly to exist among the other mothers attending as guests. When mothers share their experience and expertise at a baby shower, they are finding connections among themselves and exhibiting the intense solidarity that a pregnant woman gains as she passes into motherhood. Interestingly, this suggests that motherhood itself could be considered a condition of liminality. Recognized as not children themselves, but still identified *with* children—so that a traditional baby shower for a pregnant woman echoes a birthday party for a child—mothers have uncertain status as adults. In contrast, fathers appear to be recognized as unambiguously adult, as evidenced in the adult-like parties given when men become invited to coed or mixed baby showers. Linked as motherhood is with childhood, mothers presumably achieve their new status only when their children come into their own (if in fact this ever happens).

While baby showers are expressions and experiences of community, it is important to note the disagreements and differences that can mark them. They include the behind-the-scenes conflicts that both Megan and Audra had with family members and friends who were supposed to assist in the planning and hosting of the shower. (Both women complained to me that they had taken charge of mailing the invitations themselves.) Given the number of guests attending both Megan's and Audra's showers, instant bonds did not always form among them. In fact, drawn from the pregnant woman's circles of family members, friends, co-workers, and neighbors, the guests themselves brought differing beliefs and values about motherhood and childhood to the long tables in the reception halls where the showers were held. The work shower was particularly a site and source of discomfort for some women in my study. Although some women described their co-workers as "like family," others admitted that they might have preferred to keep work "strictly professional." While grateful for the show of kindness, some women thought that the shower might be an imposition on co-workers who had to participate, lest they appear uncaring and rude. Typically, a female co-worker who either shares a friendship with the pregnant woman or who plays a supporting role in the workplace, such as a receptionist or secretary, organizes the shower by arranging for a cake and other food and drink, and collecting money for a gift. One woman in my study expressed concern about unfairness. Because she was a supervisor in her workplace, her co-workers might feel compelled to contribute to the gift. "I am in a higher income bracket than most of the people that I work with," she explained, "and the idea that they're all going to help me get set up in my life with the baby makes me kind of uncomfortable."

Except for the work shower, most men in my study had not ever attended a shower as a guest, and not all of them were included in the baby showers given for their partners. Including men at baby showers, however, is becoming more common. The integration of men is a sign of changing expectations and experiences of fatherhood and fathering. In public discourse, the terms "parent" and "parenting" now replace "mother" and "mothering" (in addition to "father" and "fathering") in ways that appear both to describe and prescribe men's roles and responsibilities in reproduction. "Gone are the days when Dad's job was simply to keep his daughters well dressed and his sons straight. Today's fathers change diapers and brush hair, pack lunches, and bandage scraped knees. The ideal father is no longer the stern patriarch or distant provider, but a warm and accessible caregiver" (Reed 2005: 1). American middle-class men today participate in the birth and are involved in the pregnancy. Invited as guests to the baby shower, men can share their experience and expertise of fatherhood. Included alongside his partner at their baby shower, a man is recognized as an expectant father. As pleased and touched by the show of care and concern from their family members and friends as they were, however, the men who spoke with me did not necessarily attach it with the same kind of significance as women do. None could say, like Audra, that the shower was as important for them as the wedding. Even when couples were given a nontraditional co-ed or mixed baby shower, it was meaningful as the social recognition of an expectant mother.

A Grammar of Baby Things

Baby showers recognize mothers and fathers through the giving and receiving of things for the baby or for a parent to use in caring for a baby. These things communicate particular ideas and practices concerning mothers and fathers (or parents) and children. "Unlike the hand-knitted clothing of yesteryear, most of the gifts in today's baby showers are products of considerable technological sophistication. As such, they constitute a sort of grammar of modern baby-raising techniques, communicating not only the love with which they are given, but also cultural and individual notions about the appropriate roles of mother, father, and child in relation to one another" (Davis-Floyd 1992: 37). A gift of bottles and a breast pump symbolizes a mother's roles as a nurturer and as a provider, with responsibilities that include not only breastfeeding, but also earning a salary or wage. A cloth baby carrier, given to a man, represents expectations about his hands-on involvement as a father. Baby toys today include not only plush animals in pastel colors, which through their material qualities (soft, small, and cute) stand for the babies themselves, but also mobiles that play Mozart to soothe the baby, and plastic "activity centers" for the crib and other educational toys that are said to stimulate the senses.

When gifts are given and received at a baby shower, they are intended to equip a woman with all the right stuff for motherhood and mothering. Significantly, the stuff communicates what kind of mothering is considered "right." "As a whole arena of new activities, roles, and behaviors presents itself to the mother-to-be, products (their exchange and acquisition) become the key means through which types of mothering are constructed and negotiated" (Clarke 2004: 56). Returning briefly to the matter of gift registries discussed above, this is a reason why they seem helpful for both the givers and receivers of gifts. To give a breast pump and bottles to a woman who either plans to breastfeed exclusively or does not anticipate breastfeeding past the first few days or weeks with the baby might be unappreciated or misunderstood as an imposition or a judgment on the mother. The items that a woman includes on her registry in effect signal the type of mother that she envisions being.

Not only are there "bad" mothers and "good" mothers, but there is also further contestation within the category of good mothering, which is on display at the baby shower through the grammar of baby things given and received. This was especially striking at nontraditional showers, where the focus was supposed to be on people, but things still mattered. The gifts that I saw given at the nontraditional showers included special pillows designed to support breastfeeding mothers and infants, cloth slings or other carriers that maintained close physical contact between adult and child, and a gift certificate for an area diaper service. These gifts stood for a particular style of parenting and especially mothering that in the United States today is considered nontraditional, but that a number of women and men in my study valorized as a return to the tried and true. For them, breastfeeding, baby-wearing, and cloth diapering represented what is called "attachment parenting," which they described as more "natural" and "holistic" and better for the baby and "for the earth" than "modern" methods. However, pregnant women were not uncritical of attachment parenting, recognizing it as more specifically *maternal* attachment and what Hays (1996) has called "intensive mothering." Pregnant women whom I interviewed all recognized the demands that it placed particularly on mothers to be always available and to prioritize their children's wants over their own needs. Although attachment parenting represented, for women and men in my study, a rejection of commercialism and materialism, it still required things, like cloth diaper covers and baby food mills, in its practice.

At sonograms, I had observed the intense interest of pregnant women, their partners, and other family members in learning the "gender" of the baby.[2] A woman accompanying her pregnant daughter-in-law and son to the scan had wondered aloud whether they would want figure skates (for a girl) or hockey skates (for a boy). Gender matters in terms of people and things, and things matter in terms of people and gender. At traditional showers, like Audra's and Megan's, guests told me that knowing the baby's sex was necessary for knowing what things to give as gifts. Audra had not announced that she was expecting a girl, and a guest at her shower told me that she had felt "frustrated" with shopping because most baby products today, including "generic" things like bottles, come in pink or blue. Megan, who let family members and friends know that she was expecting a boy, received little tracksuits and overalls decorated with trucks. At nontraditional, coed or mixed showers, I observed an emphasis on "gender-neutral" ideas and practices concerning parents and children. In addition to things like cloth baby carriers that mothers or fathers could use, gifts included children's books and plush animals. The clothing given and received as gifts came in simple styles and colors other than the traditional pink-for-a-girl or blue-for-a-boy. Yellow and green were popular gender-neutral hues. This was true even when (or especially when) the sex of the baby was known. Rebecca and Tim had shared the news with their friends that they were expecting a boy, and the name that they had chosen for him. The name itself became the focus for the guests, as it not only marked the baby's sex, but it also made him a particular individual. The cake served at the shower was decorated with a row of small chocolate candies forming the first letter of the baby's name.

Women and men in my study described two categories of baby things—"stuff" and "gear"—which reflect the division of labor and the stereotypes associated with gender in the United States. *Stuff* referred generally to smaller, less expensive items such as clothing, toys, and instruments used in baby care, such as nail clippers and bulb aspirators. Women shopped for stuff, and gave and received it at traditional baby showers. Stuff is fleeting and frivolous in that babies outgrow things like clothing and toys, which then need to be replaced. Stuff also can be improvised easily, as I know well from my own children's rejection of teething toys for wooden spoons from the kitchen. In contrast, *gear* referred to larger, more expensive, and more technologically sophisticated items such as strollers, cribs, and car seats. Gear is necessary. As more than one couple reminded me about car seats, you cannot take a baby home from the hospital without one.

Gear also included and sometimes especially seemed to concern men. On the one hand, shopping for baby gear—that is, selecting the particular brand or color to be specified in a gift registry—involved both women and men. Couples described shopping for gear together because these were the "big" and "important" items that they saw as an "'investment" for the child, whether it was purchased by them or by family members or friends as gifts. However, men assumed primary responsibility for assembling such items as cribs and strollers. They read advice and product reviews in books like *The Baby Bargains Book* and on Web sites like babycenter.com. Men called it "research," but in fact, they shopped, which has been considered a female activity and a practice of mothering. The use of the term *gear,* rooted in other masculine pursuits, such as hunting and sports, also re-creates shopping as a male activity. As a form of "providing" for the child, it also fits into both traditional and modern fathering.

In shopping for gear, women and men in my study applied logic similar to shopping for a car, which also has been regarded stereotypically as a male activity. "Buying an expensive stroller is a lot like buying a car, with test-ride programs and glossy brochures," journalist Caitlin Flanagan suggests in *The New Yorker* magazine. "This appeals to dads, who are eager to talk about suspension and han-

dling" (2004: 46–47). In fact, cars themselves are advertised today as
a kind of baby gear, with the minivan now an icon of the American
middle-class family (Descartes and Kottak 2008). The car is an especially significant example of gear, as it is an expensive item of household consumption, and is considered among American middle-class
women and men a display of their style, taste, and status. Women
and men alike identified safety as their top priority, which is consistent with ideas about the responsibilities of parents (and fathers
especially). Dana had traded in her two-door Honda Civic, which in
her words was "compact" and "economical," for a "spacious" and
"luxurious" Subaru Forester that is regarded also as a safe and practical vehicle for winter in Michigan. The child's comfort, the adult's
convenience, and the price followed as concerns. Amanda and her
husband, Phil, sold his pick-up truck and then bought a Volkswagen
station wagon. She talked enthusiastically about their new station
wagon because they could "load it with gear" for the baby. It was
evident, however, that other considerations of taste also mattered.
Elizabeth and Ethan, poking fun at themselves, told me they had
moved "to the dark side" when they acquired a minivan. They cited
the minivan's safety first, then its capacity to hold things and people
as the reasons that they brought it home. "We are not minivan people," Ethan told me.

In a study of English middle-class women (and men), Miller (2004
[1997]) places stuff and gear for the baby in the context of the other
things that adults acquire as consumers. Without children, couples
spend money on clothing, house décor, and restaurants. With the
birth of a child, or while still awaiting its arrival, he notes "considerable concern that the material culture associated with the infant
should represent the stylistic aspirations of the parent" (2004[1997]:
36). Today, it is possible for American middle-class women and men
to choose for their children the same brands that they buy for themselves. Many makers of clothing and shoes for adults, like The Gap
and Nike, now produce lines for infants and children. A Jeep-brand
stroller is intended to appeal to Jeep drivers. It is not only that parents see children as extensions of themselves, but also that parents
regard shopping for their children as expression of their love. Manufacturers and retailers, recognizing this, have broadened the range
of baby things they make and sell. Car seats and feeding chairs now
come upholstered in navy blue and olive plaids bearing the signature
of Eddie Bauer, an outfitter of outdoor clothing and equipment. The
New York Times reports that upscale designers, too, have discovered
a small but lucrative market of women and men with seven-figure

incomes shopping for modernist cribs and changing tables and nursery themes based on Mondrian paintings. "Contemporary design for kids is really contemporary design for adults who have procreated" (Weil 2004: 74).

At the same time that the style and taste of adults are represented and reproduced in things for children, adults themselves are partaking in childlike wonder and play—indirectly, by buying new and novel playthings that they enjoy through their children's delight, and directly, by purchasing not only things like video games for themselves but also experiences "for the whole family" like Disney World vacations. In addition to favorite children's books, toys remembered from their own childhoods were gifts that women and men in my study especially enjoyed giving and receiving. A number of couples, like Elizabeth and Ethan, also favored wooden toys for older children, like building blocks, puzzles, and trains. The taste for "old" or "classic" toys is based not only on individual experiences of being children, but also on collective nostalgia for childhood as a simple, unchanging, and timeless time, far removed from adult reality. Women and men in my study could recount happy childhoods— or, if not, happier adulthoods—which inspired them to want the same or better for their children. They saw their roles as parents and responsibilities in parenting as providing and provisioning this kind of childhood. Things for the child, then, stand for children and childhood, and for the capabilities of adults as parents.

Historian Gary Cross (2004) emphasizes the significance of consumption as a practice of American middle-class parenting. "Earlier beliefs in the child's capacity for seeing the delights of nature took on new meanings when those delights became the pleasures of encountering a fantastic world of new goods and entertainments. Inevitably, childhood wonder and spending on kids became the same thing" (Cross 2004: 15). American middle-class parents today, however, are expected to participate in their children's wonder and play. They also expect it for themselves. "Many adults admire the freedom of youth and turn it into a lifestyle rather than a life stage" (Cross 2004: 15). Recapturing the freedom of youth has become an appeal made to men as fathers, especially, in advertisements. A television commercial for Disney World, for example, portrayed the transformation of a middle-aged businessman into an overgrown boy romping and splashing with his children in the Magic Kingdom.

Advertisements long have traded on images of children and infants to sell their products, even goods like soup or soap that are not necessarily connected to childhood. Increasingly, however, advertisements make their appeals directly to children themselves, by-passing adults and in particular mothers, who previously had been regarded as the shoppers of and for the family. Economist Juliet Schor contends that "children have become conduits for the con-sumer marketplace into the household, the link between advertiser and the family purse" (2004: 11). Cook (2003) links the develop-ment of American children's consumer culture during the twentieth century with changes in the discourse on fetuses and persons. He observes that the American child today has come to be seen as "an individuated, knowing consumer replete with pre-existent, natu-ralized desires and the increasing social right to realize and express them" (Cook 2003: 117). The effects of this new understanding of the American child have been far reaching. Cook contends that "the practices and institutions built up around this child-consumer laid the cultural, philosophical, and epistemological groundwork for the secular acceptance of the idea that the unborn is always and al-ready a person, the needs of which superseded those of the mother" (2003: 117). Today, it is not only that the images of children, infants, and even fetuses (in the form of sonograms) are used to advertise products to adults, or that products are advertised directly to chil-dren. In both, Cook observes "a change toward privilege the *view-point* of the child, making it the basis of authority and action" (2003: 121, emphasis in original).

In the early 1990s, a magazine advertisement for the automaker Volvo featured a sonogram image and a line of text that read: "Is something inside you telling you to buy a Volvo?" (Taylor 1992). In the early 2000s, a television commercial for Honda portrayed a couple talking with a doctor during the woman's sonogram. The fe-tus becomes animatedly engaged in the adults' conversation about cars, and gives a thumbs-up at the mention of the Odyssey minivan. Engrossed in their conversation, however, the adults in the com-mercial fail to take notice of the fetus's actions, which are the focus for the audience viewing it on television. This commercial, which women and men in my study had brought to my attention, illus-trates exactly the challenges that American feminists face in taking seriously both the importance of reproductive rights and the mean-ing that women themselves attach to pregnancy. "So long as the mother remains positioned as a mere vehicle, a vehicle for life as well as a vehicle for exchange value, she is thereby set up to be re-defined as an obstacle to life (and to consumption) by anyone or any interest that claims a moral authority to speak on behalf of those who cannot speak for themselves" (Cook 2003: 127–8).

Thanks from the Womb

In the later months and weeks of pregnancy, the "fact" of a baby becomes taken almost for granted. Rituals like the baby shower publicly acknowledge a pregnant woman and her partner as an expectant mother and father, and the giving and receiving of things symbolize the social recognition of a new baby. While all of the women and men in my study agreed on the importance of the baby shower as a ritual, they disagreed on its particular meanings, such as whether the shower was "about" the pregnant woman and expectant mother or the child. Dana, who had asked her friends for gifts of time and help, stressed its significance *for her* as an experience of community. Other women emphasized the shower as a "welcome" for the baby. Megan's guests received cards inviting them to the "Baby Stanley Shower," which identified the child with his last name. Audra's guests were invited to the "Baby B. 2003 Celebration." ("B." was the first letter of the name that Audra and her husband had chosen for their child.)[3] It also was not uncommon for the guests themselves to attach to their gifts a card or note that was addressed to the baby.

At their showers, both Megan and Audra distributed party favors as tokens of gratitude *from their babies*. Megan's favors were small, perfumed soaps in the shape of yellow duckies.[4] Each was wrapped in a yellow net bag and tied with a pastel blue ribbon, in keeping with Megan's chosen color theme. Attached to the bag was a small tag with this message: "Thank you for coming to the shower. I can't wait to meet you! Love, Dylan." Guests attending Audra's shower had received small goody bags as they entered the reception hall. Contained in the bag were a few candies, a pen for completing the word puzzles that were part of the shower games, and a laminated bookmark with this message:

> I'm sorry I couldn't be with you, but I'm terribly busy as you can see.
>
> I'm painting my eyes, cheeks, and hair. I want my Mommy and Daddy to be proud of me.
>
> Don't worry, I'll be here really soon. Be sure to come over and see me. I'll try to be looking my best.
>
> Just give Mom & Dad enough time to feed me and to see that I'm properly dressed.
>
> Thank you very much for your gift and sharing in this special day. Friendships are so hard to measure,
>
> but something Mommy and Daddy truly treasure

is this day with you.

See you soon,

Baby B.

In addition, not long after their showers, both Megan and Audra wrote and mailed letters of thanks, which they signed on behalf of their husbands and their babies. In parentheses after her own name, Megan had added "Baby Dylan-To-Be."

Initially, I had read the addressing of cards, gifts, and favors to and from the baby as simply anthropomorphizing a fetus. However, this seems a rather incomplete and impoverished misunderstanding when we take seriously the importance and meaning of an imagined or expected child to a pregnant woman, her partner, and the others who constitute their family and community. Parkin has suggested that "a person lacks a fixed, decontextualized essence but is made through a social interaction and by taking on the meaning of things standing in a special relationship to him or her" (1999: 314). Layne (2003, 1999) suggests that babies become made through the giving and receiving of gifts, which transfer the material qualities of the things to the child that is expected. However, I suggest this is not a simple relationship from "real" to "imagined" persons. The things circulating around a baby shower complicatedly reflected the pregnant woman, the imagined or expected child, and the guests at a baby shower, all of whom shift between giving and receiving.

It is meaningful that Megan especially delighted in the duckie soaps that she had found for favors. They were both baby-like and boy-like, reflective of the baby. They also were anticipated to appeal to the female guests attending the shower, reflecting the kinds of persons that both Megan and her guests were supposed to be. Distributing favors for guests to take home is a common practice at wedding receptions and other celebrations in the United States, including the goody bags (also called loot or treat bags) given at children's birthday parties. Favors are given (and thank you notes written) in part because guests expect it, and hosts consider it a custom they must follow to be polite and proper. Women like Megan and Audra also considered favors to add a "fun," "creative," and "personal" touch to their showers. Included with Megan's and Audra's favors were messages expressing the pregnant woman's gratitude, but assuming the expected child's "voice." While the expressions of gratitude themselves were sincere, their voicing through the baby is intended to be "cute" and "funny" for the guests.

Voicing through the baby also solves a few interesting cultural and social problems that the baby shower presents. For Megan and Audra in particular, issuing invitations "from" the baby and writing thank you notes on its behalf resolved the issue of not being "officially" the hosts of the shower, but still having certain responsibilities of the hosts. Both women had been more involved in planning their showers than they might have liked, and both complained to me about having had to address and stamp the invitations themselves. Voicing through the baby deflects attention from the baby shower as a celebration for the pregnant woman to the child that is imagined and expected. It enables women to receive a "shower" of gifts and even specify on a registry the things that ought to be given and received as gifts without the risk of being perceived as selfish or demanding—both traits that good mothers especially ought not to have—because the things are for the baby.

The written messages of thanks communicated the care and concern that Megan and Audra wished to reciprocate. They also did this on behalf of their husbands, performing important kin work that kept open the possibility of ties among male family members and friends (DiLeonardo 1987). They exhibited the manners of the women themselves, and in doing so, they demonstrated the capabilities that they brought to motherhood. These were women with proper manners and appropriate sentiments, which they also could teach to their children. Baby B.'s message even called attention to her Mom and Dad's training on grooming and appearance in addition to their feeding and properly dressing her. Significantly, the messages represented the particular abilities of the women to assume their children's viewpoint, which appear almost above all else to define "good" mothering for American middle-class women and men. What characterizes the language behavior of American middle-class mothers, Ochs and Schieffelin (1984) observed, is their high degree of involvement in communicating about and especially *for* their children. The messages illustrate that, as Ochs suggested, "through her own language behavior, 'mother' has become invisible" (1992: 355).

The baby shower is overladen with importance and meaning. As a ritual of ordinary pregnancy, it involves the giving and receiving of things that stand for many people and the relationships between and among them. The baby shower is the public acknowledgement and social recognition of a pregnancy, an expectant mother and father, and a child. As such, it accomplishes cultural and social work of significance for American middle-class women and men.

Notes

1. In a church wedding, for example, separation is observed when the bride's father accompanies her down the aisle and "hands" her to the groom. Transition occurs with the exchange of wedding rings and vows. Reintegration is marked with the pronouncement of the newly wed husband and wife and their recession up the aisle together.
2. From the perspective of anthropology, what was learned at the sonogram was the biological sex of the baby. However, women and men in my study, including sonographers, used "sex" and "gender" interchangeably, and preferred the term "gender" because they considered it "more polite."
3. I use pseudonyms to refer to all individuals in this study, including the children.
4. Lotte Larsen Meyer (2006) traces the cultural significance of "rubber duckies," noting that toy yellow ducks, associated with children's play, and not more realistic renderings of baby ducks, representing nature, have become symbols of infancy and childhood.

CONCLUSION
POSTPARTUM

Ordinary pregnancy "ends" in childbirth. Nicole and Betsy birthed their babies at home, as they had hoped. Betsy and Kevin, her husband, called their daughter Corazon (Spanish for "heart") a reminder of her birth on Valentine's Day. They added that the placenta also had been shaped like a heart, a detail that even the midwives themselves mentioned to me. Rebecca and Elizabeth told me that they had given birth during unexpected summer storms. Elizabeth's husband, Ethan, claimed that when their daughter arrived, the storm suddenly cleared and left a rainbow in its wake, which several friends and neighbors in the area had seen also. Brett called me to reschedule an interview that we had planned to record because she and her husband, Michael, were in the middle of painting the walls in their living room. Three days later, she called to tell me that after finishing the task, she had begun to labor. Now, she was at home with her son. Dana labored almost three days before she gave birth to her daughter. Greta broke a tooth as she bore down and pushed, working hard to birth her daughter and avoid a forceps delivery. Kerri and Amanda had Cesarean births, which had disappointed their hopes for a natural birth. Both women took comfort in the support that they received from their husbands, midwives and doulas, family members, and friends. Even with strong social support, and with the preparations she had made, becoming informed and advised on pregnancy and childbirth, Kerri said not much could have prepared her for feeling so physically and psychologically overwhelmed as she was. "Baby blues" sound cute, she said, but postpartum depression is not.

Several weeks after the birth of her son, Heather recalled for me her discharge from the hospital. She described herself as high from the birth itself, happy to have the baby safely arrived, and hectic with gathering clothing and other things, his and hers, to take home. Coming off the elevator in the lobby to await her husband, who was retrieving their car from the parking lot, Heather lifted the unfamiliar weight of the infant carrier. "I stumbled—slightly—but I stumbled," she said. Suddenly, she felt a catch in her throat and before she could stop herself, began to sob. Then, as Heather told me, the elevator doors closed behind her.

Legends and myths of larger-than-life figures, imagined and real, typically begin with stories about their births, which are supposed to tell us about their characters and their destinies. Occasionally, stories even describe the hero's time in the womb as a sign of an extraordinary personality. The future Buddha is said to have been "ablaze with light to the point that his mother's womb shone with brilliance and the outside world could see him seated therein" (Sasson 2009: 56). These stories seldom are told to illustrate or illuminate the qualities of the women who bore, then birthed the heroes. I have come to recognize how the telling of stories of pregnancy and childbirth today represents a kind of revolution for women. Sitting with Betsy in her home, now the birthplace of her daughter, or with Dana, or with Kerri, who spoke with me honestly about her postpartum depression, or with the other women whose stories I had the privilege of hearing, it became clear that these women were the heroes of their own—and their children's—stories. Their pregnancy and childbirth stories have affected me profoundly as an anthropologist, a feminist, a woman, and a mother. Until I began this study, the only stories about pregnancy and childbirth I had heard were my mother's stories about her three children. However, because she claimed that there had been nothing remarkable about her pregnancies, she also claimed not to have much to tell. In fact, I think there is much to understand about the experience of ordinary pregnancy.

In this book, I have argued for the significance of the ordinary as a framework to reorient the anthropological study of reproduction, which to date has been examined primarily in terms of medicalization, technologization, and disruption. Here, I have been interested in developing a more complicated and complete understanding of women's (and men's) own expectations and experiences of reproduction, which include the incorporation of medicine and technology *into* the practices of everyday life. Recognizing that the ordinary is as prescriptive as it is descriptive—that it is a claim that excludes and includes individuals and groups—necessitates a consideration of the larger contexts and conditions of everyday lives.

Based on ethnographic research in the United States, this book describes and discusses the ordinary pregnancies of American middle-class women. The ordinary practices of pregnancy that I examined here especially emphasized literacy and consumption. I suggest that the more expansive conceptualization of literacy and of text introduced and developed here might prove productive in studies of reproduction especially as it concerns the cultivation of sentiment and habit. Notably, being and becoming a mother entails accommodating and adopting a child's point of view. Approaching pregnancy as a literacy event underscores the cultured and socialized nature of reproduction in addition to the gendered and classed ideas and practices that constitute our lived experiences. What do pregnant women feel and how do they come to feel these feelings? How do they also make sense and meaning of the bodily sensations that reproduction induces? By calling attention to the cultivation of sentiment and habit in *selves,* it is possible also to look beyond the notion of policing *by others.*

This book also contributes to the scholarship on reproduction that particularly explores its relationship with consumption. While much of that work has been on the consequences of a consumerist ideology of "choice" for the reproductive "rights" of women, in this book, I have maintained a focus on how and why things matter to people and the significant cultural and social work that the exchange of gifts accomplishes in the making of babies and mothers.

In sum, my goal in writing this book has been to think about what ordinary pregnancy is all about—the making of a baby, the making of a mother—and to understand our expectations and experiences as culturally particular and historically peculiar. We make and remake culture and society through our lived experiences. In addition, my purpose has been to demonstrate the insight that we gain from attending—sympathetically and seriously—to what women and men do and say in their everyday lives. If we are to recognize both the importance of women's reproductive integrity and the meaning that we attach to the hope, aspiration, and imagination of a child, then this is how we might begin.

BIBLIOGRAPHY

Alexander, Greg, and Milton Kotelchuck. 2001. "Assessing the Role and Effectiveness of Prenatal Care: History, Challenges, and Directions for Future Research." *Public Health Reports* 116: 306–16.

American College of Obstetricians and Gynecologists, Committee on Obstetric Practice. 2010. "Moderate Caffeine Consumption During Pregnancy." *Committee Opinion* 462, August.

Amis, Debby, and Jeanne Green. 2002. *Prepared Childbirth—The Family Way.* Plano, TX: The Family Way Publishers.

Apple, Rima D. 2006. *Perfect Motherhood: Science and Childrearing in America.* New Brunswick, NJ: Rutgers University Press.

Arms, Suzanne. 1994. *Immaculate Deception II.* Berkeley, CA: Celestial Arts.

Armstrong, Elizabeth M. 2000. "Lessons in Control: Prenatal Education in the Hospital." *Social Problems* 47(4): 583–605.

————. 2003. *Conceiving Risk, Bearing Responsibility: Fetal Alcohol Syndrome and the Diagnosis of Moral Disorder.* Baltimore: Johns Hopkins University Press.

Bachelard, Gaston. 1994. *The Poetics of Space.* Boston: Beacon Press.

Bailey, Rebecca. 1992. "Clothes Encounters of the Gynecological Kind: Medical Mandates and Maternity Modes in the USA, 1850–1990." In *Dress and Gender: Making and Meaning,* ed. Ruth Barnes and Joanne Eichler. New York: Berg.

Baquedano-Lopez, Patricia. 2004. "Literacy Practices Across Learning Contexts." In *A Companion to Linguistic Anthropology,* ed. Alessandro Duranti. Oxford: Blackwell.

Barthes, Roland. 1980. *Camera Lucida: Reflections on Photography.* New York: Hill and Wang.

Becker, Gay. 2000. *The Elusive Embryo: How Women and Men Approach New Reproductive Technologies.* Berkeley: University of California Press.

Bessett, Danielle. 2010. "Negotiating Normalization: The Perils of Producing Pregnancy Symptoms in Prenatal Care." *Social Science and Medicine* 71: 370–77.

Bouquet, Mary. 2000. "The Family Photographic Condition." *Visual Anthropology Review* 16(1): 2–19.

———. 2001. "Making Kinship, with an Old Reproductive Technology." In *Relative Values: Reconfiguring Kinship Studies,* ed. Sarah Franklin and Susan McKinnon. Durham, NC: Duke University Press.

Bradley, Robert. 1981[1965]. *Husband-Coached Childbirth,* 3rd edition. New York: Harper and Row.

Brandt, Allen M., and Paul Rozin, eds. 1997. *Morality and Health.* New York: Routledge.

Brewis, Alexandra. 2011. *Obesity: Cultural and Biocultural Perspectives.* New Brunswick, NJ: Rutgers University Press.

Bridges, Khiara M. 2011. *Reproducing Race: An Ethnography of Pregnancy as a Site of Racialization.* Berkeley: University of California Press.

Brody, Jane. 2009. "Updating a Standard: Fetal Monitoring." *New York Times,* 7 July. http://www.nytimes.com/2009/07/07/health/07brod.html (accessed 29 May 2012).

Calhoun, Ada. 2012. "The Criminalization of Bad Mothers." *New York Times Magazine,* 25 April. http://www.nytimes.com/2012/04/29/magazine/the-criminalization-of-bad-mothers.html (accessed 25 June 2012).

Carrier, James, and Josiah Heyman. 1997. "Consumption and Political Economy." *Journal of the Royal Anthropological Institute,* N.S., 3(2): 355–73.

Carsten, Janet. 1997. *The Heat of the Hearth: The Process of Kinship in a Malay Fishing Community.* Oxford: Oxford University Press.

Cecil, Rosanne, ed. 1996. *The Anthropology of Pregnancy Loss: Comparative Studies in Miscarriage, Stillbirth, and Neonatal Death.* New York: Berg.

Chin, Elizabeth. 2001. *Purchasing Power: Black Kids and American Consumer Culture.* Minneapolis: University of Minnesota Press.

Clarke, Alison. 2001. "The Aesthetics of Social Aspiration." In *Home Possessions: Material Culture Behind Closed Doors,* ed. Daniel Miller. New York: Berg.

———. 2004. "Maternity and Materiality: Becoming a Mother in Consumer Culture." In *Consuming Motherhood,* ed. Janelle Taylor, Linda Layne, and Danielle Wozniak. New Brunswick, NJ: Rutgers University Press.

Cook, Daniel Thomas. 1995. "The Mother as Consumer: Insights from the Children's Wear Industry, 1917–1929." *Sociological Quarterly* 36(3): 505–22.

———. 2003. "Agency, Children's Consumer Culture and the Fetal Subject: Historical Trajectories, Contemporary Connections." *Consumption, Markets, and Culture* 6(2): 115–32.

Craven, Christa. 2010. *Pushing for Midwives: Homebirth Mothers and the Reproductive Rights Movement.* Philadelphia: Temple University Press.

Cross, Gary 2004. *The Cute and the Cool: Wondrous Innocence and Modern American Children's Culture.* Oxford: Oxford University Press.

Cunningham, Clark. 2000. "Foreword." In *Beyond Kinship: Social and Material Reproduction in House Societies,* ed. Rosemary Joyce and Susan Gillespie. Philadelphia: University of Pennsylvania Press.

Curtis, Glade, and Judith Schuler. 2008. *Your Pregnancy Week by Week,* 6th edition. New York: Da Capo Press.

Davis-Floyd, Robbie. 1992. *Birth as an American Rite of Passage.* Berkeley: University of California Press.

———. 1994. "Mind over Body: The Pregnant Professional." In *Many Mirrors: Body Image and Social Relations,* ed. Nicole Sault. New York: Routledge.

DeCasper, Anthony, and Melanie Spence. 1986. "Prenatal Maternal Speech Influences Newborns' Perception of Speech Sounds." *Infant Behavior and Development* 9: 133–50.

Declercq, Eugene, Carol Sakala, Maureen P. Corry, and Sandra Applebaum. 2006. *Listening to Mothers II: Report of the Second National U.S. Survey of Women's Childbearing Experiences.* New York: Childbirth Connection.

Declercq, Eugene, Carol Sakala, Maureen P. Corry, Sandra Applebaum, and Peter Risher. 2002 *Listening to Mothers: Report of the First National U.S. Survey of Women's Childbearing Experiences.* New York: Maternity Center Association.

DeLoache, Judy, and Alma Gottlieb. 2000. *A World of Babies: Imagined Childcare Guides for Seven Societies.* New York: Cambridge University Press.

Descartes, Lara, and Conrad P. Kottak. 2008. "Patrolling the Boundaries of Childhood in Middle-Class 'Ruburbia.'" In *The Changing Landscape of Work and Family in the American Middle Class: Reports from the Field,* ed. Elizabeth Rudd and Lara Descartes. New York: Lexington Books.

DeVault, Marjorie. 1991. *Feeding the Family: The Social Organization of Caring as Gendered Work.* Chicago: University of Chicago Press.

Dick-Read, Grantly. 1953[1944]. *Childbirth without Fear.* New York: Harper and Row.

DiLeonardo, Michaela. 1987. "The Female World of Cards and Holidays: Women, Families, and the Work of Kinship." *Signs* 12(30): 440–53.

Dubow, Sara. 2011. *Ourselves Unborn: A History of the Fetus in Modern America.* Oxford: Oxford University Press

Duden, Barbara. 1993. *Disembodying Women: Perspectives on Pregnancy and the Unborn.* Cambridge, MA: Harvard University Press.

———. 1999. "The Fetus on the 'Farther Shore': Toward a History of the Unborn." In *Fetal Subjects, Feminist Positions,* ed. Lynn Morgan and Meredith Michaels. Philadelphia: University of Pennsylvania Press.

Ehrenreich, Barbara. 1989. *Fear of Falling: The Inner Life of the Middle Class.* New York: Perennial.

Ehrenreich, Barbara, and Deirdre English. 1989. *For Her Own Good: Two Centuries of the Experts' Advice to Women.* New York: Anchor.

Eisenberg, Arlene, Heidi Murkoff, and Sandee Hathaway. 1996[1984]. *What to Expect When You're Expecting.* New York: Workman.

———. 1986. *What to Eat When You're Expecting.* New York: Workman.

England, Pam, and Rob Horowitz. 1998. *Birthing from Within: An Extra-Ordinary Guide to Childbirth Preparation.* Albuquerque, NM: Partera Press.

Farquhar, Judith, and Margaret Lock. 2007. "Introduction." In *Beyond the Body Proper: Reading the Anthropology of Material Life,* ed. Judith Farquhar and Margaret Lock. Durham, NC: Duke University Press.

Ferguson, Charles. 1977. "Baby Talk as a Simplified Register." In *Talking to Children: Language Input and Acquisition,* ed. Catherine Snow and Charles Ferguson. Cambridge: Cambridge University Press.

Fischer, Eileen, and Brenda Gainer. 1993. "Baby Showers: A Rite of Passage in Transition." *Advances in Consumer Research* 30: 320–24.

Fischer, Rachel C., Joseph B. Stanford, Penny Jameson, and M. Jann DeWitt. 1999. "Exploring the Concepts of Intended, Planned, and Wanted Pregnancy." *Journal of Family Practice* 48(2): 117.

Flanagan, Caitlin. 2004. "Annals of Retail: Bringing up Baby." *The New Yorker,* 15 November.

Gaskin, Ina May. 1977. *Spiritual Midwifery.* Summertown, TN: The Book Publishing Company.

———. 2003. *Ina May's Guide to Childbirth.* New York: Bantam Books.

Georges, Eugenia. 1997. "Fetal Ultrasound Imaging and the Production of Authoritative Knowledge in Greece." In *Childbirth and Authoritative Knowledge: Cross-Cultural Perspectives,* ed. Robbie Davis-Floyd and Carolyn F. Sargent. Berkeley: University of California Press.

Geurts, Kathryn. 2002. *Culture and the Senses: Bodily Ways of Knowing in an African Community.* Berkeley: University of California Press.

Ginsburg, Faye D., and Rayna Rapp. 1995. "Introduction: Conceiving the New World Order." In *Conceiving the New World Order: The Global Politics of Reproduction,* ed. Faye D. Ginsburg and Rayna Rapp. Berkeley: University of California Press.

Glenn, Evelyn Nakano. 1994. "Social Constructions of Mothering: A Thematic Overview." In *Mothering: Ideology, Experience, and Agency,* ed. Evelyn Nakano Glenn, Grace Chang, and Linda Rennie Forcey. New York: Routledge.

Goer, Henci. 1999. *The Thinking Woman's Guide to a Better Birth.* New York: Perigee.

Gottlieb, Alma. 2004. *The Afterlife Is Where We Come from: The Culture of Infancy in West Africa.* Chicago: University of Chicago Press.

Guttmacher Institute. 2012. "Requirements for Ultrasound." *State Policies in Brief,* 1 July.

Han, Sallie. 2008. "Seeing the Baby in the Belly: Family and Kinship at the Ultrasound Scan." In *The Changing Landscape of Work and Family in the American Middle Class: Reports from the Field,* ed. Elizabeth Rudd and Lara Descartes. New York: Lexington Books.

———. 2009a. "Seeing Like a Family: Fetal Ultrasound Images and Imaginings of Kin." In *Imagining the Fetus: The Unborn in Myth, Religion, and Culture,* ed. Vanessa Sasson and Jane Marie Law. Oxford: Oxford University Press.

———. 2009b. "'That's When I Imagine It as a Baby': Belly Talk and Reproductive Politics." *Anthropology News,* February.

———. 2009c. "Making Room for Daddy: Men's 'Belly Talk' in the Contemporary United States." In *Reconceiving the Second Sex: Men, Masculinity, and*

Reproduction, ed. Marcia Inhorn, Tine Tjornhoj-Thomsen, Helene Gold-berg, and Maruska la Cour Mosegaard. New York: Berghahn Books.

————. 2009d. "Men at Home: The Work of Fathers in the House and the Nursery." *Phoebe: Journal of Gender and Cultural Critiques* 21(2): 21–30.

Harkness, Sara, and Charles Super. 1996. *Parents' Cultural Belief Systems: Their Origins, Expressions, and Consequences.* New York: Guilford.

Harmon, Katherine. 2010. "Mother's Pregnancy Weight Linked to Child's Obesity." *Scientific American,* 5 August. http://www.scientificamerican.com/article.cfm?id=mothers-pregnancy-weight (accessed 12 July 2012).

Hays, Sharon. 1996. *The Cultural Contradictions of Motherhood.* New Haven, CT: Yale University Press.

Heath, Shirley Brice. 2001[1984]. "What No Bedtime Story Means: Narrative Skills at Home and School." In *Linguistic Anthropology: A Reader,* ed. Alessandro Duranti. New York: Wiley-Blackwell.

Henry, Linda. 2001. "What's Going on in Your Baby's Mind?" *Baby Talk,* August.

Hotchner, Traci. 1997[1979]. *Pregnancy and Childbirth,* 3rd edition. New York: Avon Books.

Howard, Vicki. 2006. *Brides, Inc.: American Weddings and the Business of Tradition.* Philadelphia: University of Pennsylvania Press.

Hulbert, Ann. 2003. *Raising America: Experts, Parents, and a Century of Advice about Children.* New York: Knopf.

Ingold, Tim. 2000. *The Perception of the Environment: Essays in Livelihood, Dwelling, and Skill.* New York: Routledge.

Inhorn, Marcia. 1994. *Quest for Conception: Gender, Infertility, and Egyptian Medical Traditions.* Philadelphia: University of Pennsylvania Press.

————. 2003. *Local Babies, Global Sciences: Gender, Religion, and In Vitro Fertilization in Egypt.* New York: Routledge.

Inhorn, Marcia, Tine Tjornhoj-Thomsen, Helene Goldberg, and Maruska la Cour Mosegaard. 2009. "Introduction: The Second Sex in Reproduction? Men, Sexuality and Reproduction." In *Reconceiving the Second Sex: Men, Masculinity, and Reproduction,* ed. Marcia Inhorn, Tine Tjornhoj-Thomsen, Helene Goldberg, and Maruska la Cour Mosegaard. New York: Berghahn Books.

Iovine, Vicki. 1995. *The Girlfriends' Guide to Pregnancy.* New York: Pocket Books.

Ivry, Tsipy. 2010. *Embodying Culture: Pregnancy in Japan and Israel.* New Brunswick, NJ: Rutgers University Press.

Jordan, Brigitte. 1992[1978]. *Birth in Four Cultures: A Cross-cultural Investigation of Childbirth in Yucatan, Holland, Sweden, and the United States.* Prospect Heights, IL: Waveland.

Joyce, Rosemary. 2000. "Heirlooms and Houses: Materiality and Social Memory." In *Beyond Kinship: Social and Material Reproduction in House Societies,* ed. Rosemary Joyce and Susan Gillespie. Philadelphia: University of Pennsylvania Press.

Keane, Webb. 1997. "Religious Language." *Annual Review of Anthropology* 26: 47–71.

Kitzinger, Sheila.1991. *Home Birth.* New York: Dorling Kindersley.

Klassen, Pamela. 2001. *Blessed Events: Religion and Home Birth in America.* Princeton, NJ: Princeton University Press.

Kukla, Rebecca. 2005. *Mass Hysteria: Medicine, Culture, and Mothers' Bodies.* Lanham, MD: Rowman and Littlefield Publishers.

Kulick, Don. 1992. *Language Shift and Cultural Reproduction: Socialization, Self, and Syncretism in a Papua New Guinean Village.* Cambridge: Cambridge University Press.

Kulick, Don, and Bambi Schieffelin. 2004. "Language Socialization." In *A Companion to Linguistic Anthropology,* ed. Alessandro Duranti. Oxford: Blackwell.

Ladd-Taylor, Molly. 2004. "Mother-Worship/Mother-Blame: Politics and Welfare in an Uncertain Age." *Journal of the Association for Research on Mothering* 6(1): 7–15.

Ladd-Taylor, Molly, and Lauri Umansky. 1998. "Introduction." In *"Bad" Mothers: The Politics of Blame in Twentieth-Century America,* ed. Molly Ladd-Taylor and Lauri Umansky. New York: NYU Press.

Lambek, Michael. 2012. "Introduction." In *Ordinary Ethics: Anthropology: Language, and Action,* ed. Michael Lambek. New York: Fordham University Press.

Lamott, Anne. 1993. *Operating Instructions: A Journal of My Son's First Year.* New York: Pantheon.

Laxton-Kane, Martha, and P. Slade. 2002. "The Role of Maternal Prenatal Attachment in a Woman's Experience of Pregnancy and Implications for the Process of Care." *Journal of Reproductive and Infant Psychology* 20(4): 253–66.

Layne, Linda L. 2000. "'He Was a Real Baby with Baby Things': A Material Culture Analysis of Personhood, Parenthood, and Pregnancy Loss." *Journal of Material Culture* 5(3): 321–45.

———. 2003. *Motherhood Lost: A Feminist Account of Pregnancy Loss in America.* New York: Routledge.

———. 2009. "The Home Pregnancy Test: A Feminist Technology?" *Women's Studies Quarterly* 37(1 and 2): 61–79.

———, ed. 1999. *Transformative Motherhood: On Giving and Getting in a Consumer Culture.* New York: NYU Press.

Lazarus, Ellen. 1997. "What Do Women Want? Issues of Choice, Control, and Class in American Pregnancy and Childbirth." In *Childbirth and Authoritative Knowledge: Cross-Cultural Perspectives,* ed. Robbie Davis-Floyd and Carolyn F. Sargent. Berkeley: University of California Press.

Leavitt, Judith Walzer. 1986. *Brought to Bed: Childbearing in America, 1750–1950.* Oxford: Oxford University Press.

Leavitt, Sarah. 2006. "'A Private Little Revolution': The Home Pregnancy Test in American Culture." *Bulletin of the History of Medicine* 80(2): 317–45.

Lewin, Ellen. 1993. *Lesbian Mothers: Accounts of Gender in American Culture.* Ithaca, NY: Cornell University Press.

————. 2009. *Gay Fatherhood: Narratives of Family and Citizenship in America.* Chicago: University of Chicago Press.

Long, Elizabeth. 2003. *Book Clubs: Women and the Uses of Reading in Everyday Life.* Chicago: University of Chicago Press.

MacDonald, Margaret. 2007. *At Work in the Field of Birth: Midwifery Narratives of Nature, Tradition, and Home.* Nashville, TN: Vanderbilt University Press.

Mansfield, Becky. 2008. "The Social Nature of Natural Childbirth." *Social Science and Medicine* 66: 1084–94.

Mardorossian, Carine. 2003. "Laboring Women, Coaching Men: Masculinity and Childbirth Education in the Contemporary United States." *Hypatia* 18(3): 113–34.

Markens, Susan. 2007. *Surrogate Motherhood and the Politics of Reproduction.* Berkeley: University of California Press.

Markens, Susan, Carol Browner, and Nancy Press. 1997. "Feeding the Fetus: On Interrogating the Notion of Maternal-Fetal Conflict." *Feminist Studies* 23(2): 351–72.

Martin, Emily. 1992[1987]. *The Woman in the Body: A Cultural Analysis of Reproduction.* Boston: Beacon Press.

————. 1997. "The Egg and the Sperm: How Science Has Constructed a Romance Based on Stereotypical Male-Female Roles." In *Situated Lives: Gender and Culture in Everyday Life,* ed. Louise Lamphere, Helena Ragone, and Patricia Zavella. New York: Routledge.

Martin, Joyce, Brady E. Hamilton, Paul D. Sutton, Stephanie J. Ventura, Fay Menacker, and Sharon Kirmeyer. 2006. "Births: Final Data for 2004." *National Vital Statistics Reports* 55, no. 1 (29 September). US Department of Health and Human Services, Centers for Disease Control and Prevention.

Matthews, Sandra, and Laura Wexler. 2000. *Pregnant Pictures.* New York: Routledge.

McDonnell, Jane Taylor. 1998. "On Being the 'Bad' Mother of an Autistic Child." In *"Bad" Mothers: The Politics of Blame in Twentieth-Century America,* ed. Molly Ladd-Taylor and Lauri Umansky. New York: NYU Press.

McKeown, Thomas. 2010[1978]. "Determinants of Health." In *Understanding and Applying Medical Anthropology,* ed. Peter J. Brown and Ron Barrett. New York: McGraw Hill.

Meyer, Lotte Larsen. 2006. "Rubber Ducks and Their Significance in Contemporary American Culture." *Journal of American Culture* 29(1): 14–23.

Michaels, Meredith, and Lynn Morgan. 1999. "Introduction: The Fetal Imperative." In *Fetal Subjects, Feminist Positions,* ed. Lynn Morgan and Meredith Michaels. Philadelphia: University of Pennsylvania Press.

Miller, Daniel. 1998. *A Theory of Shopping.* Ithaca, NY: Cornell University Press.

————. 2004[1997]. "How Infants Grow Mothers in North London. In *Consuming Motherhood,* ed. Janelle Taylor, Linda Layne, and Danielle Wozniak. New Brunswick, NJ: Rutgers University Press.

Mintz, Sidney W. 1986. *Sweetness and Power: The Place of Sugar in Modern History.* New York: Penguin Books.

————. 1997. *Tasting Food, Tasting Freedom: Excursions into Eating, Power, and the Past.* Boston: Beacon Press.

Mitchell, Lisa. 2001. *Baby's First Picture: Ultrasound and the Politics of Fetal Subjects.* Toronto: University of Toronto Press.

Montemurro, Beth. 2005. "Add Men, Don't Stir: Reproducing Traditional Gender Roles in Modern Wedding Showers." *Journal of Contemporary Ethnography* 34(1): 6–35.

Moore, Mignon R. 2011. *Invisible Families: Gay Identities, Relationships, and Motherhood among Black Women.* Berkeley: University of California Press.

Morgan, Lynn. 1997. "Imagining the Unborn in the Ecuadorian Andes." *Feminist Studies* 23(2): 323–50.

————. 2006[1990]. "When Does Life Begin? A Cross-cultural Perspective on the Personhood of Fetuses and Young Children." In *Talking about People: Readings in Cultural Anthropology,* ed. William Haviland, Robert Gordon, and Luis Vivianco. New York: McGraw Hill.

————. 2009. *Icons of Life: A Cultural History of Human Embryos.* Berkeley: University of California Press.

Mullings, Leith. 1995. "Households Headed by Women: The Politics of Race, Class, and Gender." In *Reconceiving the New World Order: The Global Politics of Reproduction,* ed. Faye D. Ginsburg and Rayna Rapp. Berkeley: University of California Press.

Nader, Laura. 1972. "Up the Anthropologist: Perspectives Gained from Studying Up." In *Reinventing Anthropology,* ed. Dell Hymes. New York: Pantheon Books.

Neergaard, Lauran. 2009. "Is Your Toddler's Vocabulary Thiiis Big?" *Los Angeles Times,* 22 February. http://articles.latimes.com/2009/feb/22/news/adna-toddlers22 (accessed 6 July 2012).

Nichter, Mimi. 2000. *Fat Talk: What Girls and Their Parents Say about Dieting.* Cambridge, MA: Harvard University Press.

Oakley, Ann. 1984. *The Captured Womb: A History of the Medical Care of Pregnant Women.* Oxford: Blackwell.

Oaks, Laury. 2001. *Smoking and Pregnancy: The Politics of Fetal Protection.* New Brunswick, NJ: Rutgers University Press.

Ochs, Elinor. 1992. "Indexing Gender." In *Rethinking Context: Language as an Interactive Phenomenon,* ed. Alessandro Duranti and Charles Goodwin. Cambridge: Cambridge University Press.

Ochs, Elinor, and Bambi Schieffelin. 1984. "Language Acquisition and Socialization: Three Developmental Stories and Their Implications." In *Culture Theory: Essays on Mind, Self, and Emotion,* ed. Richard Shweder and Robert Levine. Cambridge: Cambridge University Press.

O'Reilly, Andrea. 2004. "Introduction." In *Mother Outlaws: Theories and Practices of Empowered Mothering,* ed. Andrea O'Reilly. Toronto: Women's Press.

Papen, Uta. 2008. "Pregnancy Starts with a Literacy Event: Pregnancy and Antenatal Care as Textually Mediated Experiences." *Ethnography* 9(3): 377–402.

Parkin, David. 1999. "Mementoes and Transitional Objects in Human Displacement." *Journal of Material Culture* 4(3): 303–20.

Peel, Elizabeth. 2009. "Pregnancy Loss in Lesbian and Bisexual Women: An Online Survey of Experiences." *Human Reproduction* 25(3): 721–27.

Petchesky, Rosalind Pollack. 1987. "Fetal Images: The Power of Visual Culture in the Politics of Reproduction." *Feminist Studies* 13(2): 263–92.

Petrozza, John C., and Inna Berin. 2011. "Early Recurrent Pregnancy Loss." Medscape Reference, http://emedicine.medscape.com/article/260495-overview (accessed 29 May 2012).

Pope, Tara Parker. 2009. "Study Urges Weight Gain to Be Curbed in Pregnancy." *New York Times*, 29 May.

Rabin, Roni Caryn. 2009. "New Goal for the Obese: Zero Gain in Pregnancy." *New York Times*, 15 December. http://www.nytimes.com/2009/12/15/health/15obese (accessed 8 July 2012).

Ragone, Helena. 1994. *Surrogate Motherhood: Conception in the Heart.* Boulder, CO: Westview.

Rapp, Rayna. 1999. *Testing Women, Testing the Fetus: The Social Impact of Amniocentesis in America.* New York: Routledge.

Rasmussen, Kathleen M., and Ann L. Yaktine, eds. 2009. "Weight Gain During Pregnancy: Reexamining the Guidelines," report prepared for the Committee to Reexamine IOM Pregnancy Weight Guidelines of the Institute of Medicine and the National Research Council. http://www.iom.edu/Reports/2009/Weight-Gain-During-Pregnancy-Reexamining-the-Guidelines.aspx (accessed 8 July 2012).

Reed, Richard. 2005. *Birthing Fathers: The Transformation of Men in American Rites of Birth.* New Brunswick, NJ: Rutgers University Press.

Roberts, Dorothy. 1997. *Killing the Black Body: Race, Reproduction, and the Meaning of Liberty.* New York: Pantheon.

Rothman, Barbara Katz. 1987. *The Tentative Pregnancy.* New York: Viking.

Sandelowski, Margarete. 1994. "Separate, but Less Unequal: Fetal Ultrasonography and the Transformation of Expectant Mother/Fatherhood." *Gender and Society* 8(2): 230–45.

Sanger, Carol. 2008. "Seeing and Believing: Mandatory Ultrasound and the Path to a Protected Choice." *UCLA Law Review* 56: 351–408.

Santora, Marc. 2004. "Fetal Photos: Keepsake or Health Risk?" *New York Times*, 17 May.

Sasson, Vanessa. 2009. "A Womb with a View: The Buddha's Final Fetal Experience." In *Imagining the Fetus: The Unborn in Myth, Religion, and Culture*, ed. Vanessa Sasson and Jane Marie Law. Oxford: Oxford University Press.

Scheper-Hughes, Nancy. 1992. *Death without Weeping: The Violence of Everyday Life in Brazil.* Berkeley: University of California Press.

Schieffelin, Bambi, and Elinor Ochs. 1986. "Language Socialization." *Annual Review of Anthropology* 15: 163–91.

Schor, Juliet. 2004. *Born to Buy.* New York: Scribner.

Sears, William, and Martha Sears. 1997. *The Pregnancy Book.* Boston: Little, Brown.

————. 2003. *The Baby Book*. Boston: Little, Brown.

Simonds, Wendy. 1992. *Women and Self-Help Culture: Reading between the Lines*. New Brunswick, NJ: Rutgers University Press.

Small, Meredith. 1998. *Our Babies, Ourselves: How Biology and Culture Shape the Way We Parent*. New York: Anchor.

Solinger, Rickie. 2005. *Pregnancy and Power: A Short History of Reproductive Politics in America*. New York: NYU Press.

Stabile, Carol. 1992. "Shooting the Mother: Fetal Photographer and the Politics of Disappearance." *Camera Obscura* 28: 178–205.

Stearns, Peter. 2003. *Anxious Parents: A History of Modern Childrearing in America*. New York: NYU Press.

Street, Brian V., and Niko Besnier. 2009[1994]. "Aspects of Literacy." In *Making Sense of Language: Readings in Culture and Communication,* ed. Susan D. Blum. New York: Oxford University Press.

Strong, Thomas H. 2000. *Expecting Trouble: What Expectant Parents Should Know about Prenatal Care in America*. New York: NYU Press.

Taussig, Karen-Sue. 2009. *Ordinary Genomes: Science, Citizenship, and Genetic Identities*. Durham, NC: Duke University Press.

Tavernise, Sabrina. 2012. "Whites Account for Under Half of Births in US." *New York Times,* 17 May. http://www.nytimes.com/2012/05/17/us/whites-account-for-under-half-of-births-in-us.html (accessed 31 May 2012).

Taylor, Janelle. 1992. "The Public Fetus and the Family Car: From Abortion Politics to a Volvo Advertisement." *Public Culture* 4: 69–87.

————. 2000. "Of Sonograms and Baby Prams: Prenatal Diagnosis, Pregnancy, and Consumption." *Feminist Studies* 26(2): 391–418.

————. 2004. "A Fetish Is Born: Sonographers and the Making of the Public Fetus." In *Consuming Motherhood,* ed. Janelle Taylor, Linda Layne, and Danielle Wozniak. New Brunswick, NJ: Rutgers University Press.

————. 2008. *The Public Life of the Fetal Sonogram: Technology, Consumption, and the Politics of Reproduction*. New Brunswick, NJ: Rutgers University Press.

Taylor, Janelle, Linda Layne, and Danielle Wozniak, eds. 2004. *Consuming Motherhood*. New Brunswick, NJ: Rutgers University Press.

Teman, Elly. 2010. *Birthing a Mother: The Surrogate Body and the Pregnant Self*. Berkeley: University of California Press.

Thompson, Charis. 2007. *Making Parents: The Ontological Choreography of Reproductive Technologies*. Cambridge, MA: MIT Press.

United States Department of Health and Human Services, Office of Minority Health. 2012. "Infant Morality and African Americans." http://minorityhealth.hhs.gov/templates/content.aspx?ID=3021 (accessed 26 June 2012).

Upton, Rebecca, and Sallie Han. 2003. "Maternity and Its Discontents: 'Getting the Body Back' after Pregnancy." *Journal of Contemporary Ethnography* 32(6): 670–92.

Ventura, Stephanie J. 2009. "Changing Patterns of Nonmarital Childbearing in the United States." *NCHS Data Brief* 18 (May 2009). US Department of Health and Human Services, Centers for Disease Control and Prevention.

Walks, Michelle, and Naomi McPherson, eds. 2011. *An Anthropology of Mothering*. Toronto: Demeter Press.

Walzer, Susan. 1998. *Thinking about the Baby: Gender and Transitions into Parenthood*. Philadelphia: Temple University Press.

Weil, Elizabeth. 2004. "The Modernist Nursery." *New York Times Magazine,* 28 November.

Weiner, Annette. 1992. *Inalienable Possessions: The Paradox of Keeping While Giving*. Berkeley: University of California Press.

Wertz, Richard, and Dorothy Wertz. 1989. *Lying-In: A History of Childbirth in America*. New Haven, CT: Yale University Press.

Weschler, Toni. 1995. *Taking Charge of Your Fertility*. New York: Harper-Perennial.

Wilcox, Allen J. 1988. "Incidence of Early Loss of Pregnancy." *New England Journal of Medicine* 319(4): 189–94.

Wilson, Samantha L. 2001. "Attachment Disorders: Review and Current Status." *Journal of Psychology* 135(1): 37–51.

Wolf, Naomi. 2001. *(Mis)conceptions: Truth, Lies, and the Unexpected on the Journey to Motherhood*. New York: Anchor.

Zelizer, Viviana. 1985. *Pricing the Priceless Child: The Changing Social Value of Children*. Princeton, NJ: Princeton University Press.

INDEX